DISEASES

OF

POVERTY

GEISEL SERIES IN GLOBAL HEALTH AND MEDICINE

Series editors:

Lisa V. Adams, MD, associate professor of medicine and associate dean for global health at Geisel School of Medicine at Dartmouth

John R. Butterly, MD, professor of medicine at Geisel School of Medicine at Dartmouth and the Dartmouth Institute of Health Policy and Clinical Practice

This series, sponsored by Dartmouth College Press, draws on the scholarly and practical expertise of a diverse group of health care practitioners and public health professionals engaged in combatting a wide range of challenging health issues faced by low-income countries around the globe. Books in the series vary: they may focus on a geographical area, such as Central America; a specific topic, such as surgery; or a particular set of health issues in their environmental and political contexts. All books in the series should speak to medical students, health care and public health professionals, and anyone interested in engaging in global health work or learning more about the issues and problems facing our global society.

For a complete list of books that are available in the series, visit www .upne.com

Kathleen Allden and Nancy Murakami, editors, *Trauma and Recovery on War's Border: A Guide for Global Health Workers*

Lisa V. Adams and John R. Butterly, *Diseases of Poverty: Epidemiology, Infectious Diseases, and Modern Plagues*

Margo J. Krasnoff, editor, *Building Partnerships in the Americas: A Guide for Global Health Workers*

Anji E. Wall, *Ethics for International Medicine: A Practical Guide for Aid Workers in Developing Countries*

Kate Tulenko, *Insourced: How Importing Jobs Impacts the Healthcare Crisis Here and Abroad*

Laurel A. Spielberg and Lisa V. Adams, editors, *Africa: A Practical Guide for Global Health Workers*

John R. Butterly and Jack Shepherd, *Hunger: The Biology and Politics of Starvation*

DISEASES

OF

POVERTY

Epidemiology,
Infectious Diseases,
and Modern Plagues

LISA V. ADAMS AND
JOHN R. BUTTERLY

DARTMOUTH COLLEGE PRESS
Hanover, New Hampshire

Dartmouth College Press
An imprint of University Press of New England
www.upne.com
© 2015 Trustees of Dartmouth College
All rights reserved
Manufactured in the United States of America
Designed by Vicki Kuskowski
Typeset in Bembo by A. W. Bennett Book Composition

For permission to reproduce any of the material in this book, contact Permissions,
University Press of New England, One Court Street, Suite 250, Lebanon NH
03766; or visit www.upne.com

Library of Congress Cataloging-in-Publication Data
Adams, Lisa V., author.
Diseases of poverty : epidemiology, infectious diseases, and modern
plagues / Lisa V. Adams and John R. Butterly.
    p. ; cm.
Includes index.
ISBN 978-1-61168-751-4 (cloth : alk. paper) — ISBN 978-1-61168-752-1
(pbk. : alk. paper) — ISBN 978-1-61168-753-8 (ebook)
I. Butterly, John R., author. II. Title.
[DNLM: 1. Communicable Diseases—epidemiology. 2. Poverty. 3. World
Health. 4. Communicable Disease Control. 5. Public Health—methods. WA
110]
RA418.5.P6
362.1086'942—dc23
2014037197

5 4 3 2 1

We dedicate this book to our global health students and international collaborators—both have been a source of great inspiration to us over the years. —LVA and JRB

CONTENTS

CONTENTS

PROLOGUE

Dr. Agnes Binagwaho, Minister of Health, Rwanda

Every human being is born with the right to health. Because we are equal, it is unacceptable that people suffer and die simply because of where they are born. In this seminal book, you will be taken on a journey across the globe where health care delivery challenges are tackled and diseases are studied and measured. To understand global health, you must grapple with issues of equity and social justice. Indeed, in the role of a student—which I will forever consider myself to be—we have the opportunity to dive deeply into these lessons with great diligence and thoughtfulness.

To place equity firmly at the core of health care delivery requires a serious, evidence-based focus on poverty: the single most debilitating cause of suffering and unnecessary mortality across the globe. As this text will remind you, the number of purely biological causes of disease pale in comparison to the amount of illness and agony caused by inadequate infrastructure, suboptimal health worker training, lack of access to curative medicines, and so on, in other words, to determinants rooted in the context of poverty. Breaking the cycle of poverty and disease is the only way forward, and I therefore encourage you to embrace one of the key messages of this book, which is that health is beyond a health sector, or beyond health studies, for that matter. We must come to view well-being as a goal, with myriad interrelated inputs along the way from other domains, like education, economics, and engineering.

Over the course of your global health education, you should aim to gather a wide array of tools and methods of study available to you, including those that are qualitative, quantitative, ethnographic, biosocial, and epidemiological, to name a few. Learning the broader context of a health system and of disease will not only aid you in your career, but it will also enable you to become a good partner to the people, communities, and countries you work alongside. This book presents an important venue through which to study and understand examples of when partnerships and programs have succeeded, fallen short, or failed.

In my country of Rwanda, we aimed to interlink the objectives of health and economic growth through our economic development and poverty reduction strategy, within which health is considered a tenet of growing our nation's economy. Over the past twenty years, through this measure and by guaranteeing health as a human right within our constitution, we have, alongside our partners, been able to double life expectancy since the 1994 genocide. Mortality due to tuberculosis and malaria has plummeted, and child and maternal mortality have both been halved. We have begun to address the burden of cancer, cardiac disorders, diabetes, and other diseases considered by some to be too complex to tackle in low-income countries. In 2012, our national human papillomavirus vaccination program covered 93 percent of our girls, who now can live without fear of dying unnecessarily from cervical cancer. I mention these milestones not only to illustrate the power of community-driven, equity-focused, partnership-supported, nationally owned programs, but I also share this to illuminate the potential and potency of ambition and hope. In 1995 after the genocide, it was almost impossible to imagine a Rwanda like it is today: with 45,000 community health workers, a state-of-the-art pathology lab on the site of what had been a military base, forty-two district hospitals dotting the map in even distribution. But some did have that imagination, and our shared progress to date reflects such optimism.

Today the world faces two distinct narratives. For some of us, great progress in improving health outcomes has been registered despite economic constraints. This is because we were able to make great strides in the response to HIV/AIDS, malaria, tuberculosis, and other major killers, all accomplishments of which were unthinkable two decades before. But for others, they may argue that nothing has really changed given that health disparities are still far too great across the world and within a country's own border. From my point of view, both narratives are right. We have indeed made dramatic advancements toward health equity, and yet so much remains to be done. This is where you come in. Today the world is a better place than yesterday, even if so much remains on our plate. You are the ones who will be charged with pushing the agendas of bigger dreams and aspirations in global health. Never forget that there is no plan too ambitious and no target out of reach if the right methods are applied. Remind yourself that pessimism only leads to paralysis. Young students around the world give us great hope, with their boundless optimism and a hunger for change.

By honestly and intensively engaging with this material, you join the thousands throughout the world who are fighting every day for better health for all, because each human being deserves the best. Critical to this fight are the true, long-term partnerships that are built around shared values, equity, science, local ownership direction, participation of all stakeholders, sustainability, and the country's evidence-based context—epidemiological, political, and economic. I encourage you to connect and partner with your peers and your mentors in different contexts and countries to take on some of the world's biggest problems together.

There are innumerable roles for those who wish to contribute to the field of global health. The world needs cardiologists, architects, computer technicians, dosimetrists, professors, medical anthropologists, businesspeople, social workers, politicians, pharmacists, and so forth. I have no doubt that readers of this book will go on to make an impact in their individual ways. And the key to this impact is understanding advancement as being achieved through partnership and collaboration, such that the contributions of infectious disease clinicians are synergistic with those of supply chain managers, and that the goodwill of donors is synergistic with needs of places and countries.

As a student or practitioner of global health, one of the most important jobs you have at this time is to listen well, immerse yourself deeply in an issue, and learn to find your voice. It is an everyday mindset change and behavioral exercise. Never think you need to travel many miles—by train, boat, or plane—to participate in and act for improving global health. It is not about people from high-income countries coming to have internships or work in low-income countries. Rather, it is about all the sick and destitute in the world who are suffering, and about your readiness to engage this knowledge with cultural humility no matter where you are today. Start in your community where you live, work, and learn, because global health starts where any human being is standing. It starts in the room in which you find yourself today.

Never forget the importance and privilege of serving. Never be shy about adding your contributions to the fight for health equity. We need your sharp mind and your hopefulness in this fight, and we challenge you to challenge the status quo. You must cherish this opportunity throughout your studies, work, and this text, and you must walk away with the mindset that each and every citizen of the world inherited his and her right to health, and it is our global imperative to fulfill that right.

DISEASES

OF

POVERTY

1

INTRODUCTION TO GLOBAL HEALTH

Lisa V. Adams, John R. Butterly, and Hoiwan Cheung

It is easier to build strong children than it is to repair broken men.

—Frederick Douglass

Poverty is not an accident . . . it is man-made and can be removed by the actions of human beings.

—Nelson Mandela

WHAT IS GLOBAL HEALTH?

Global health has recently emerged as its own academic discipline. While many definitions of global health have been put forward, we endorse the definition offered by Koplan et al. in *The Lancet*: "global health is an area for study, research, and practice that places a priority on improving health and achieving equity in health for all people worldwide." [1] They further write, "global health emphasizes transnational health issues, determinants, and solutions; involves many disciplines within and beyond the health sciences and promotes interdisciplinary collaboration; and is a synthesis of population-based prevention with individual-level clinical care." This aspirational definition captures the core aspects of global health as an inclusive approach to health and public health that lives at the intersection of many different disciplines. Attacking any global health issue requires critical thinking and a clear framework of how outcomes are defined, how parameters will be measured,

1

and, most importantly, what the goals of a project are before delving into the delicate details.

GLOBAL HEALTH CHALLENGES: COMPLEX AND MULTIFACTORIAL

Within global health practice, those from different disciplines bring their own lens or perspective to global health challenges. Colleagues in infectious disease may participate in global health through work to prevent the development of drug-resistant strains of major communicable diseases, while epidemiologists may focus their efforts on studies of disease burden, data that are critical in defining public health priorities and interventions. A government public health official may choose to promote education programs that encourage healthy behaviors or increased utilization of vaccinations, or might work to improve sanitation systems in the poorest communities. A health services researcher may promote the standardization of "best practices" in medicine and health care delivery, while an environmentalist might feel that environmental pollution, resource depletion, and global warming are the most fundamental issues to be addressed.

GLOBAL HEALTH SOLUTIONS: MULTIDISCIPLINARY AND COLLABORATIVE

Throughout these varied approaches and activities, there are common threads that link them together: the belief that health is a shared responsibility that transcends geographical, cultural, and man-made barriers, and the recognition that the health of individuals, populations, and our planet are inextricably linked. This is a novel idea considering how much societal, cultural, religious, and legal rules differ from person to person, community to community, state to state, and nation to nation. But despite these differences, providing everyone with the *opportunity* to live a full, generally healthful life and to reach their full potential is a universally held goal.

To clarify further, we must consider a change in paradigms. A more forward concept of global health requires that we no longer accept that the health of individuals is limited by countries or geographic separation within the modern world; it is the concept that the health of people globally is interconnected in a way not possible before travel and communication technologies that allow us to be half a world away within twelve hours (or virtually face to face with another individual within seconds). In the face of these facts, *global health is the recognition that the health of an individual is no longer insulated from the health states of others and that health is now a shared responsibility within a global community* Thus, as global health advocates, we have an obligation to pool our resources to help others live a healthful life in accordance with the World Health Organization's definition of health: a state of complete physical, mental, and social well-being, not simply a life free from disease or disability. [2]

Why Should You Care about Global Health?

There are a number of reasons that global health should also be every individual's concern, regardless of his or her level of involvement with the medical community:

1. We live in an increasingly globalized world, one in which we are no longer protected from diseases that arise in other nations.
The speed with which diseases can spread due to the ease of global travel, variability in immunization rates for different populations, and increasing resistance to available antimicrobial therapies has increased the size of susceptible populations. Very few locations remain in the world where populations are completely insulated

from the outside world. In the past, mountains, deserts, and oceans kept diseases from spreading, but this is no longer the case.

As a result, infectious diseases that arise in one country have a much higher probability of affecting the health of populations in other countries. Poor public health conditions or policies, including poor sanitation, insufficient health education, the overuse of antibiotics, or close contact with domestic animals, can give rise to new disease pathogens, multidrug-resistant forms of common diseases, or increasing prevalence of known diseases. In other words, technically advanced populations that are insulated from the risks associated with living in an environment of poor public health measures and limited infrastructure are now more directly connected to populations in which increasingly virulent, resistant organisms can evolve and flourish.

For a relevant case study, examine the 2003 SARS pandemic that started in the Guangdong province of China. In the end, this disease infected over eight thousand people and took the lives of more than seven hundred (average fatality rates approached 10 percent, similar to those seen in cholera epidemics). The virus arose by jumping from wildlife to humans (zoonotic transmission), most likely as a result of close contact between humans and wildlife in Asian markets. [3] By the end of the year, hundreds of cases were documented in Taiwan, Korea, and Canada, with cases spreading to a total of twenty-five countries outside of China and Taiwan. The Chinese government responded by developing and enforcing strong regulations within China's wildlife markets, preventing the further spread of the virus.

In the SARS example, Chinese health policy affected the development and subsequent worldwide spread of a novel virus, one for which we have no vaccine. While the government did ultimately impose new policies related to the use of wildlife for food, they initially failed to report the epidemic, thereby allowing the virus to spread beyond their borders. The lessons learned in this case emphasize how important it is for us to recontextualize global health and coordinate responses to emerging infectious diseases.

2. Investing in health will go a long way.
The downstream effects of poor health can result in shorter lifespans, increasing disability, lower wages, lower productivity, increased costs, and lower quality of life. [4–8] Thus, health is an investment that will yield benefits that far outweigh the initial costs. For example, a parent who becomes blind from cataracts will have a harder time remaining in the work force and earning a steady and sufficient income to feed his or her family. If a young child suffers from malnutrition, evidence suggests that in addition to having poorer health outcomes, that child will have fewer educational achievements, lower income, and a lower standard of living, and will make less of a contribution to the society in which he or she lives. [9] Investing in the health of individuals is also an investment in a country's future GDP, economy, average income, standards of living, and, most importantly, *human capital* for the future.

3. Advancing equality in health is both ethically and economically the right thing to do.
As the WHO definition implies, health allows individuals to take advantage of their human potential. Limiting investments in human capital, such as education, also limits the number of innovative ideas and the ability to execute them. Investments in education can increase a country's economic growth, but these investments will likely fall short of their potential if individuals are in poor health and unable to perform at their best, or access to education is limited by gender or economic status.

Additionally, creating ties with the rest of the world will create a global community with more partner nations by investing in a cause on which we can all agree. By interacting more with other nations on a shared vision of improving health, and by understanding that one actually pays a price if another is not well (and receives a benefit if others are well and performing at their full potential), we will gain much more through the sharing of culture, innovation, and community.

We should spend some time reflecting on the opportunities we were given in our lives and the factors that contributed to our successes. Recognize that we are not all self-made individuals. Give back by passing on to others the chance to have more opportunities to live a healthy and productive life.

This book has two primary goals. First, it aims to present global health not as a topic solely defined in medical terms, but in a broader sense using the ultimate human determinants of ecological and biological health: economics, education, infrastructure, culture, and personal liberty. This approach will be applied to the main infectious causes of the greatest morbidity and mortality worldwide. While we acknowledge that noncommunicable diseases are contributing to an increasing proportion of death and disease even in the poorest countries, here we will focus on communicable diseases in the first of a planned two-volume series on global health. This intentional focus leads to the second purpose of this book, which is to provide a primer in the basic biology of the infectious diseases responsible for the majority of preventable deaths in developing nations; the history and science of disease epidemiology; specific examples of successes and failures at disease control and eradication; special issues of particularly vulnerable groups (women and children); and the sociocultural, political, and health-system issues involved in each of these.

Only a few decades ago, we were ready to declare a victory over infectious diseases. Today, infectious diseases, generally considered as diseases associated with poor public health infrastructure, are responsible for significant morbidity and mortality throughout the world. Even resource-rich countries are plagued by resistant "super bugs" and antibiotic misuse despite sophisticated infrastructure aimed at limiting exposure to the usual pathogens. This book will examine the epidemiology and social impact of past and present infectious disease epidemics in the developing and developed world. Lessons from past and current efforts to control global infectious diseases will guide our examination of the high-profile infectious disease pathogens poised to threaten our health in the future. Looking toward the future, the growing impact of chronic diseases, the diseases of affluence, such as hypertension, diabetes, obesity, and cardiovascular disease, will be addressed as well. This book is intended for nonmedical professionals who want an overview of some of the critical challenges in global health. Global health is one means by which we are linked to our fellow humans; we think this connection should drive us to action to address these challenges to achieve the lofty goal of health and well-being for all.

ADDRESSING THE WORLD'S CHALLENGES: THE MILLENNIUM DEVELOPMENT GOALS

The devastation and unprecedented human suffering caused by World War II had a sobering effect on the leaders of what at the time was referred to as the First World (originally this term referred to countries allied with the United States, while the Second World countries included the Soviet Union and their allies). Third World countries were "undeveloped" countries, not yet aligned. Since the end of the Cold War, the First World countries have been those with highly developed economies and social infrastructure, while Third World countries have been those with poorly developed economies, minimal infrastructure, and a substantial percentage of their population living in extreme poverty. A number of organizations, including the United Nations and the World Health Organization, were founded at the end of World War II as a direct response to the need for global collaboration around multiple issues; among these were the issues of human rights and international codes of conduct between sovereign nations. As part of this mandate, the United Nations established a Commission of Human Rights charged with creating a document intended to be an International Bill of Rights. A broadly representative group, chaired by Eleanor Roosevelt, produced the document, which was eventually adopted by the General Assembly of the United Nations on December 10, 1948, and known as the Universal Declaration of Human Rights. Recognized as the first global acknowledgment of rights to which all human beings are entitled, it consists of a preamble and thirty articles. Specifically relevant to the topic of this book is Article 25, which reads:

- Everyone has the right to a standard of living adequate for the health and well-being of himself and of his family, including food, clothing, housing and medical care and necessary social services, and the right to security in the event of unemployment, sickness, disability, widowhood, old age or other lack of livelihood in circumstances beyond his control.
- Motherhood and childhood are entitled to special care and assistance. All children, whether born in or out of wedlock, shall enjoy the same social protection. [10]

This document, founded in sound, noncontroversial ethical principles, was non-binding. Not surprisingly, and despite substantial effort by many notable world leaders over the ensuing decades, the world described in this document has yet to be realized. In terms of global health, the Millennium Development Project (http://www.unmillenniumproject.org/) and the related Millennium Development Goals (http://www.un.org/millenniumgoals/) represent the international community's renewed commitment to end extreme poverty and the associated human suffering. This renewed commitment by nearly two hundred nations reflects the growing realization by governments, economists, universities, and thought leaders in all walks of life that we live in a global community, that the health and well-being of every one of us is inextricably linked to that of our fellow members of the human race, that the nations that recognize this interdependence and develop the means to actively engage in the global community will be those that succeed in the next iteration of human history.

THE MILLENNIUM DEVELOPMENT GOALS

There are eight Millennium Development Goals, each with one or more associated targets to be achieved. In reading them, you will see how each relates to the universal human rights guaranteed to all members of our global society sixty-five years ago.

Considerable progress has been made in reaching many of the goals established. The goal of halving the proportion of the world's population living in extreme poverty has been reached, two billion people have achieved sustainable access to safe drinking water, significant gains have been attained in reducing mortality rates from malaria and tuberculosis, with a 25 percent decrease in mortality from malaria and an estimated twenty million lives saved from tuberculosis. Progress has, however, not been made uniformly for all the goals, and there remain geographical disparities that require refocusing of resources and energy. While the percent of the world's population that is undernourished has decreased from 23.2 percent in 1990–1992 to 14.9 percent in 2010–2012, one-eighth of the world's population (12.5 percent or 900 million people by the time you are reading this) remains chronically undernourished, and, in an apparent paradox, it is estimated that 7 percent of the world's children under the age of five years are overweight (one-quarter of these children live in sub-Saharan Africa). We are lagging in our efforts to provide access to antiretroviral therapy for those with HIV/AIDS; access to primary education, especially in rural areas;

BOX 1-1

Goal 1: Eradicate Extreme Hunger and Poverty

Target 1. Halve, between 1990 and 2015, the proportion of people whose income is less than $1 a day.

Target 2. Halve, between 1990 and 2015, the proportion of people who suffer from hunger.

Goal 2: Achieve Universal Primary Education

Target 3. Ensure that by 2015, children everywhere, boys and girls alike, will be able to complete a full course of primary schooling.

Goal 3: Promote Gender Equality and Empower Women

Target 4. Eliminate gender disparity in primary and secondary education, preferably by 2005, and in all levels of education no later than 2015.

Goal 4: Reduce Child Mortality

Target 5. Reduce by two-thirds, between 1990 and 2015, the under-five mortality rate.

Goal 5: Improve Maternal Health

Target 6. Reduce by three-quarters, between 1990 and 2015, the maternal mortality ratio.

Goal 6: Combat HIV/AIDS, Malaria, and Other Diseases

Target 7. Have halted by 2015 and begun to reverse the spread of HIV/AIDS.

Target 8. Have halted and begun to reverse the incidence of malaria and other major diseases.

Goal 7: Ensure Environmental Stability

Target 9. Integrate the principles of sustainable development into country policies and programs and reverse the loss of environmental resources.

Target 10. Halve by 2015 the proportion of people without sustainable access to safe drinking water and basic sanitation.

Target 11. Have achieved by 2020 a significant improvement in the lives of at least one hundred million slum dwellers.

BOX 1-1 (CONT.)

Goal 8: Develop a Global Partnership for Development

Target 12. Develop further an open, rule-based, predictable, non-discriminatory trading and financial system (includes a commitment to good governance, development, and poverty reduction, both nationally and internationally).

Target 13. Address the special needs of the Least Developed Countries (includes tariff- and quota-free access for Least Developed Countries' exports, enhanced program of debt relief for heavily indebted poor countries [HIPCs], cancellation of official bilateral debt, and more generous official development assistance for countries committed to poverty reduction).

Target 14. Address the special needs of landlocked developing countries and small island developing states (through the Program of Action for the Sustainable Development of Small Island Developing States and 22nd General Assembly provisions).

Target 15. Deal comprehensively with the debt problems of developing countries through national and international measures in order to make debt sustainable in the long term.

Target 16. In cooperation with developing countries, develop and implement strategies for decent and productive work for youth

Target 17. In cooperation with pharmaceutical companies, provide access to affordable essential drugs in developing countries.

Target 18. In cooperation with the private sector, make available the benefits of new technologies, especially information and communications technologies. [2]

and resolution of gender disparities. [11] There is yet much to accomplish. Understanding the nature of the problems faced—the science of epidemiology, infectious disease and the specific diseases faced; the public health issues associated with inadequate social infrastructure; the role of the many governmental agencies and nongovernmental organizations (NGOs)—will make your work in the global health arena more effective and hopefully more rewarding.

As this book neared publication, the world's attention was on the tragic Ebola outbreak in West Africa. First diagnosed in early December 2013, it took many months before the international community recognized Ebola as a major crisis, and the World Health Organization declared it "a public health emergency of international concern." [12] In the countries with cases, existing poor health system infrastructure, including a lack of infection control practices in clinical settings facilitated transmission of the virus. Case numbers rose at a frightening rate with projections reaching one million cases by January 2015. [13] Associated with a 60 percent mortality rate, this was everyone's worst nightmare for a contagious disease outbreak. Transmission of Ebola to two u.s. healthcare workers caring for a patient in Texas revealed our own system's vulnerabilities. Some subsequent reactions were extreme, fostering fear and hysteria rather than sound and reasonable public health practices.

As international response starts to gather momentum, we are seeing a decrease in Ebola incidence. Simultaneously, researchers are working to identify therapeutic agents and a vaccine at a pace rarely possible in drug and vaccine development. This crisis shines a light on important themes of this book: the interconnectedness of our global population and the devastating role that poverty and weak health systems have on local and global populations. The sooner we start effectively collaborating to address these challenges, the sooner we will see extreme poverty and the associated diseases be controlled, eliminated and eventually eradicated.

REFERENCES

1. Koplan JP, Bond TC, Merson MH, Reddy KS, Rodriguez MH, Sewankambo NK, et al. Consortium of Universities for Global Health Executive Board. Towards a common definition of global health, *Lancet.* 2009 Jun 6;373(9679):1993–5.

2. Preamble to the Constitution of the World Health Organization as adopted by the International Health Conference, New York, 19–22 June, 1946; signed on 22 July 1946 by the representatives of 61 States (Official

Records of the World Health Organization, no. 2, p. 100) and entered into force on 7 April 1948.

3. Yardley J. After its epidemic arrival, SARS vanishes. *New York Times*. 2005 May 15.

4. Contoyannis P, Rice N. The impact of health on wages: Evidence from the British Household Panel Survey. *Empirical Economics*. 2001/11/01;26(4):599–622.

5. Smith JP. Healthy bodies and thick wallets: the dual relation between health and economic status. *The Journal of Economic Perspectives*. 1999;13(2):145–66.

6. Boles M, Pelletier B, Lynch W. The relationship between health risks and work productivity. *Journal of Occupational and Environmental Medicine*. 2004;46(7):737–45.

7. Goetzel RZ, Hawkins K, Ozminkowski RJ, Wang S. The health and productivity cost burden of the "top 10" physical and mental health conditions affecting six large US employers in 1999. *Journal of Occupational and Environmental Medicine*. 2003;45(1):5–14.

8. Wilson IB, Cleary PD. Linking clinical variables with health-related quality of life. *JAMA: the Journal of the American Medical Association*. 1995;273(1):59–65.

9. Galler JR, Bryce C, Waber DP, Zichlin ML, Fitzmaurice GM, Eaglesfield D. Socioeconomic outcomes in adults malnourished in the first year of life: a 40-year study. *Pediatrics*. 2012 Jul;130(1):e1–7. PubMed PMID: 22732170. Pubmed Central PMCID: PMC3382923. Epub 2012/06/27. eng.

10. United Nations Universal Declaration of Human Rights, Article 25: December 10, 1948.

11. United Nations Statistics Division, Millennium Development Goals Indicators. http://unstats.un.org/unsd/mdg/Host.aspx?Content=Products/ProgressReports.htm, accessed on September 6, 2013.

12. WHO Ebola Response Team. Ebola virus disease in West Africa—the first 9 months of the epidemic and forward projections. *N Engl J Med*. 2014 Oct 16;371(16):1481–95.

13. Meltzer MI, Atkins CY, Santibanez S, Knust B, Petersen BW, Ervin ED, Nichol ST, Damon IK, Washington ML; Centers for Disease Control and Prevention (CDC). Estimating the future number of cases in the Ebola epidemic—Liberia and Sierra Leone, 2014–2015. *MMWR Surveill Summ*. 2014 Sep 26;63 Suppl 3:1–14.

2

GLOBAL HEALTH

Systems, Agencies, Organizations, and Other Stakeholders

Lisa V. Adams

Numerous organizations and agencies are engaged in some aspect of global health work. While it is impossible to discuss all of them, this chapter provides an overview of the types of entities involved in this work and the common, though not exhaustive, forms their work may take. We include a brief historical review of the global health agencies and institutions that were formed during the twentieth century, as they were the precursors to the key global health agencies that exist today. To understand the roles of the various stakeholders, it will be important to be familiar with the structure of health systems outside the United States as well. This will provide the context for the often complicated and crowded stage of global health actors.

STAKEHOLDERS IN GLOBAL HEALTH

If asked to make a list of the stakeholders in global health, it might include a range of nongovernmental organizations (NGOs), governmental agencies, universities, health care workers, and patients, among others. We can classify these entities into broad categories such as donor, governmental or nongovernmental, international or national agencies, policy makers, think tanks, businesses, researchers, and technical assistance agencies. As the list under each head-ing grows, it becomes necessary to consider how all these entities interact with each other.

In terms of donor assistance, one major distinction is between foreign aid entities that provide bilateral versus multilateral assistance. Bilateral assistance is essentially direct aid from one government to, or for the benefit of, one or more other governments. For example, when the u.s. government provides assistance to one or more countries for a specific project or program, this is considered bilateral assistance. This type of aid tends to be very content- and donor-driven, with the specifics of the project or goals determined by the donor. The President's Emergency Plan for AIDS Relief, announced by President George W. Bush during his 2003 State of the Union address and now known by its acronym PEPFAR, is an example of bilateral assistance. This program provides support for the treatment and prevention of HIV infection to fifteen high HIV-prevalence countries. Compare this form of aid with multilateral assistance, which is indirect assistance provided by multiple donor governments, usually without any stipulations, to multilateral organizations that then in turn provide assistance to one or more countries on behalf of the donors. An example of multilateral assistance is the u.s. government's payments to the World Health Organization, the World Bank, or The Global Fund to Fight AIDS, Tuberculosis and Malaria. This organization then provides assistance to multiple countries without donor-determined conditions attached. Multilateral assistance is an effective means of extending the reach of every participating donor by leveraging resources. In contributing to a multilateral agency, the donor delegates to the multilateral agency the responsibility for setting priorities, selecting recipients, distributing funds, and monitoring outcomes. There are also hybrids of multilateral/bilateral assistance that cross over and involve some multilateral and some bilateral aspects of aid.

A simple and straightforward framework to help distinguish bilateral from multilateral agencies is that multilateral agencies tend to be agencies of the United Nations such as the World Health Organization (WHO), the United Nations Children's Fund (UNICEF), and the United Nations High Commission for Refugees (UNHCR). The World Bank is another multilateral agency. Bilateral agencies are typically a specific aid program, or an arm of the government that provides unilateral assistance. In the United States, it is the United States Agency for International Development (USAID), which is under the State Department. Similarly, Canada has its Canadian International Development Agency and the United Kingdom has its Department for International Development.

There are numerous nonprofit agencies and many nongovernmental organizations (NGOs), several of which you will recognize and may have supported in the past: Oxfam, CARE, and Médecins Sans-Frontières/Doctors Without Borders, for example. In addition to these international NGOs, there are many national NGOs in low- and middle-income countries that are the common recipients of international aid. Some prominent examples are the Bangladesh Rural Advancement Committee (BRAC) in Bangladesh or the Haitian Group for the Study of Kaposi's Sarcoma and Opportunistic Infections (GHESKIO) in Haiti. These are names that you might not be familiar with unless you have worked in those countries. Needless to say, some of the national NGOs tend to be highly effective and do excellent work. Both national and international NGOs come in all sizes and with a range of resources; some have annual budgets of a few thousand dollars while others have budgets of hundreds of millions.

Next let's consider foundations and other philanthropic organizations. Some of the more prominent foundations include the Bill and Melinda Gates Foundation and the Rockefeller Foundation. Many academic institutions from the United States and Europe are involved in global health education/capacity building, research, or practice. In recent years, the groundswell of interest in global health among students has led to many institutions establishing centers, institutes, and offices of global health to coordinate and grow their activities in this area. There are also international institutions, such as Aga Khan University, which is involved in global health work outside of its home country of Pakistan. Lastly, there are for-profit agencies or contractors and businesses that are engaged in global health activities. Businesses take interest in global health for a variety of reasons: to ensure the safety and good health of their employees, as acts of good will toward the country in which they are operating, or as part of their broader corporate responsibility program. Pharmaceutical giants such as Abbott or Bristol-Myers Squibb have well-established foundations or global citizenship programs, but nonmedical companies are also involved. Examples are plentiful, and include Chevron supporting HIV prevention in Nigeria and Intel devoting resources to educating girls and women.

HISTORY OF GLOBAL HEALTH ORGANIZATIONS

To understand the current roles of the main organizations in global health, it will be useful to examine their history and formation. Evidence of disease is present in our earliest records of human history. Using molecular identification methods, scientists have detected diseases such as tuberculosis (TB) and malaria in the skeletal remains of the early Egyptians. [1] Early public health action was taken in response to some of the first major epidemics that occurred. One of the first recorded epidemics was that of the plague in AD 542. This was followed many years later by a second major plague epidemic, known as the "Black Death" epidemic in the fourteenth century, which is still considered the most destructive epidemic in human history. During the Middle Ages, hospitals were established in Europe. While today we may think of hospitals as places to go for specialized care and treatment, initially they primarily served an important public health purpose: to quarantine the infirm (while the term "quarantine" refers to any isolation or detention of an individual to prevent spread of disease, its derivation comes from the fact that forty days was traditionally considered the appropriate length of time for such isolation). Without understanding the details of disease transmission, medical providers did know that removing people who had contagious diseases from the community could prevent its further spread.

The sanitary reform in England, which occurred on the heels of a cholera epidemic in 1831, was the beginning of a systematic approach to public health and the creation of health boards. In 1851, the International Sanitary Conference in Paris confirmed the important role of quarantine to control epidemics of plague, cholera, and yellow fever. This marked the first international efforts to coordinate the control of diseases within a country or across country borders.

The International Sanitary Bureau was established in 1902 in Washington, D.C. This bureau, with its focus on the Western Hemisphere, was followed a few years later by the opening in 1909 of the International Public Hygiene Office, which became commonly known as the Paris Office. It was the Paris Office that began setting standards and goals for controlling epidemics, which marked the early, groundbreaking work in public health and disease prevention. Further public health efforts were thwarted, to some extent, by World War I. In 1918, toward the end of the war, the great influenza epidemic hit. In efforts to quarantine the sick, those with influenza symptoms were crowded into stadiums, auditoriums, and even airplane hangars to accommodate the large numbers. In the end, twenty million people died in that devastating outbreak.

In 1920, the League of Nations was formed in Geneva, under which the League of Nations Health Office—the precursor to the World Health Organization—was established. While this was a landmark in the history of public and global health, the period was still plagued by significant challenges. Despite the comparatively few players in global health at the time, coordination was still problematic and funding shortages were common. As happens today, global health agencies were trying to lay their claims to their particular areas, and the fight for resources was played out by fewer contenders but over a smaller pot of resources. During this time, there were simultaneous advances in science and medicine that led to our increased understanding about disease transmission and effective therapies that significantly impacted the direction and growth of the field of public health. The League of Nations Health Office and the Paris Office worked together to achieve standardization of epidemiologic data collection, dissemination of vital health statistics, publication of the Weekly Epidemiologic Record (a precursor to the CDC's Morbidity and Mortality Weekly Report), establishment of additional international offices and setting agendas and research priorities, and development of technical commissions to set standards for public health.

ESTABLISHING THE WORLD HEALTH ORGANIZATION

In 1945, the League of Nations was replaced by the United Nations (UN). As the UN was being formed, discussions began about whether there should be an associated global health organization. On April 7, 1948, the World Health Organization (WHO) was established and its constitution was enacted, and April 7 is recognized today as World Health Day to commemorate the establishment of the WHO. At the first World Health Assembly meeting, which included representation from all WHO member states, immediate priorities were set. These included malaria, women's and children's health, TB, sexually transmitted diseases, nutrition, and environmental sanitation. Interestingly, these issues remain health priorities for the world today.

The WHO has a clear and succinct mission: the attainment by all peoples of the highest possible level of health. Health is further defined as "a state of complete physical, mental and social well-being and not merely the absence of disease or infirmity." [2] Currently, the WHO is governed by 193 member states through the World Health Assembly meetings and is led by the WHO director-general, who serves five-year terms. The WHO has its headquarters in Geneva and maintains six regional offices to represent their region's health interests and priorities: African Region, Region of the Americas, Eastern Mediterranean Region, European Region, South-East Asia Region, and Western Pacific Region.

The WHO strives to achieve its mission through two primary activities. The first is to provide central technical services. Specifically, the WHO is responsible for producing international guidelines and standards to control and address outbreaks of certain diseases. It disseminates information including educational materials. It standardizes vaccines and medicines; in addition to establishing the Expanded Programme of Immunizations (EPI), the WHO has developed an essential medicines list, which includes the medicines that every country should have as a bare minimum available to its population. It also produces publications and supports and promotes health research. The WHO is not a funding agency; this is often misunderstood in global health circles. The WHO actually receives funding for its activities from member state contributions and from external donors such as USAID and the Gates Foundation. It is important to note that the WHO provides support and technical assistance services to governments *only* when requested by countries to assist in tackling their public health problems. The WHO has no authority to impose their regulations or recommendations on a country. Rather, WHO technical teams work in countries where they have been invited to assist. They do not function as public health law enforcers.

Some of the most notable landmarks in the WHO's history include its launch of the EPI in the mid-1970s, followed by the creation of the essential medicines list in 1977. The WHO was also behind the 1978 Alma Ata Declaration, a document that promotes and proposes health care for all. The WHO was a major player in the smallpox eradication effort, the only successful disease eradication campaign to date. Attempting to repeat the success of smallpox eradication, the WHO has also been a leader in the polio eradication initiative, and since the start of this initiative, the number of polio cases has been reduced by 99 percent. The work of the WHO is often associated only with infectious disease control, but the WHO is also involved in noncommunicable disease control. For example, the WHO launched the Framework Convention on Tobacco Control in 2003, a major antismoking/antitobacco effort. In terms of emerging diseases, the WHO played a critical role in identifying and successfully containing the outbreak of Severe Acute Respiratory Syndrome (SARS) in 2003. Following the SARS epidemic, the WHO's roles, responsibilities, and priorities were expanded to include responding to disease outbreaks.

The priorities of the World Health Organization can thus be summarized as follows: Enhancing global health security, perhaps the foundation of its work; controlling and preventing disease outbreaks to avert crises; developing international health regulations and guidelines; trying to minimize the suffering following natural disasters and conflicts; and coordinating emergency health responses to disease outbreaks. As mentioned above, the WHO also has units devoted to preventing chronic noncommunicable diseases. The WHO is also focused on improving health care quality and access in an effort to improve the health and well-being of the world's population. And finally, the WHO's resolutions and recommendations urge adherence but never oblige members to comply.

THE ROLE OF GOVERNMENTS IN HEALTH

In most countries of the world, the government is responsible for providing health care to its citizens and managing the public health system. Outside of the United States, a country's Ministry of Health (MOH) is the body that typically organizes the health sector and services. In the United States, our Department of Health and Human Services (DHHS) is the closest analogous agency. Under the MOH, categorical or vertical disease programs tackle a particular disease of public health importance. Examples include national TB and leprosy programs, national HIV/AIDS control programs, and national malaria control programs. These programs employ health care providers, public health workers, and community health workers who focus on diagnosing and treating patients with that particular disease. This means that in some settings, a community health worker from the TB control program will visit a patient to ensure that the patient is taking their TB medicines. The worker typically would not follow up on whether the patient was properly treated for a recent episode of malaria, or whether the children in the household are up to date on their immunizations or sleeping under insecticide-treated bed nets. This is a distinct disadvantage to vertical programs and specialized staff. Recently, however, there has been greater interest in adopting a more broad-based approach to integrating care services, either by strengthening general primary care services or by linking two frequently coexisting diseases such as TB and HIV.

It is impossible to mention health-system strengthening without acknowledging the health care worker shortage most low-income countries are experiencing. Health care worker emigration has become so severe that in the last few years in more than half a dozen African countries there are as many domestically trained health care workers working outside of their country as working inside it. Obviously there are many reasons for this phenomenon—referred to as "push/pull" factors—but the reasons people leave their country to practice elsewhere are generally the same reasons any of us would do so: to seek a livable wage for themselves and their families, a safe environment in which to raise their children with decent schools to provide a good education, and opportunities for professional growth and career advancement. This is admittedly an oversimplification of this complex dynamic, but it is does capture some of the underlying reasons that contribute to the common push factors. Many countries lose their health professionals to places like the United States and Europe where a larger health care work force is needed—and actively recruited—to staff its less prestigious hospitals and health centers. And lastly, there is also the "internal brain drain" which refers to the loss of health professionals not through emigration but to positions in national and international NGOs, which removes them from clinical work to serve in administrative roles. Due in large part to unregulated salary structures between the public sector and international aid organizations, better pay (and interesting work) can be the lure for an English-speaking health care worker to leave his or her clinical job for a position with an NGO.

In the United States, the DHHS is the government's "principal agency for protecting the health of all Americans." [3] The DHHS oversees many important offices and services, such as the Centers for Disease Control and Prevention (CDC, the leading U.S. public health agency), the Food and Drug Administration, and the National Institutes of Health. In the global health sphere, the Office of Global Affairs (also under DHHS) serves as the United States's global liaison for setting global health priorities and building relationships with foreign MOHs and other multilateral partners overseas. In addition, Peace Corps volunteers, who are primarily placed in rural areas, often work on health-related activities.

UNITED STATES AGENCY
FOR INTERNATIONAL DEVELOPMENT

The United States Agency for International Development (USAID), under the State Department, is one of the most important actors on the global health stage. USAID was created by an executive order in 1961 by President Kennedy. With the Marshall Plan to rebuild Europe ending roughly ten years earlier, there was great interest in finding the best means to continue providing assistance to countries in need. The 1961 Foreign Assistance Act reorganized U.S. foreign aid programs and made an important distinction by separating military and nonmilitary aid. USAID was thus not placed under the Department of Defense, but rather under the Department of State. Currently, USAID works in more than a hundred countries and spends a tiny fraction, less than 1 percent, of the federal budget.

Generally speaking, the purpose of U.S. foreign assistance is twofold. First, it is to further American foreign policy interests in expanding democracy and free markets and second, and hopefully not less importantly, it is to improve the lives of citizens in the developing world. Looking at today's headlines, we can find many examples in which our foreign assistance plans and activities mirror or are closely linked to our foreign policy interests in the world. In other words, our U.S. foreign assistance arena is just another stage on which our policy interests and the existing imbalances of power and resources are played out. Needless to say, this impacts everything from our foreign relations to our prioritization of activities and policies. USAID has transitioned its focus over the past five decades from a focus on ensuring basic human needs, to stabilizing foreign financial systems, to sustainable development and democracy building, to the most recent focus on rebuilding governments, infrastructure, and civil society in Iraq and Afghanistan.

Global health has been defined as one of the key program areas of USAID (the others being agriculture and food security; democracy, human rights, and governance; economic growth and trade; education; ending extreme poverty; environment and global climate change; gender equality and women's empowerment; science, technology, and innovation; water and sanitation; and working in crisis and conflict). [4] USAID assists countries under certain circumstances: when recovering from disaster, trying to escape poverty, and when engaged in democratic reform. Its headquarters is in Washington, D.C., and it is divided into bureaus both by geographic area and by sector. The sectors correspond to the key program areas listed above and its geographic regions are Africa, Asia, Latin America and the Caribbean, and Europe and Eurasia. Thus there is some intentional overlap in the program and geographic areas, for example, someone in the African bureau may cover health programs while someone in the global health bureau may work in some African countries. USAID also has mission offices in many countries where it is active. Mission offices are semiautonomous and support the intentional shift in recent years to move more of the decision making closer to the communities being served. Many mission office positions are filled with program and project managers from the host country, which adds local expertise. A country mission office will have its own budget for programs; it will define its own priorities and work in relationship with the Washington headquarters, but it will make many of the programmatic decisions for that country.

USAID provides competitively awarded contracts to different organizations, mostly NGOs but also to some U.S. government agencies such as the CDC and U.S. Public Health Service. An increasingly common mode of operating is the awarding of large grants to a consortium of organizations where a prime recipient organization serves as the coordinating agency and will subcontract with various partners to provide the needed technical expertise. This approach shifts much of the administrative burden and management of the grant and its activities to the primary recipient organization. USAID also provides technical assistance and capacity building, especially in global health programming.

In recent years, there have been increasing criticisms over the "militarizing" of U.S. foreign aid, the increasing overlap between military and humanitarian assistance. For example, it was the U.S. military that distributed the food aid in Somalia in the 1990s, and the Department of Defense has played a major role in providing humanitarian assistance in Iraq and Afghanistan. Overlap in the roles of military and aid workers can create confusion and poorly coordinated activities or, worse, place aid workers at increased risk. In a 2009 letter to North Atlantic Treaty Organization (NATO) delegates signed by more than fifteen NGOs, the authors urged NATO troops to clearly identify themselves in Afghanistan and distinguish military actions from humanitarian activities. [5] Not doing so, they argued, placed Afghan civilians and aid workers at risk because the Afghan military forces would not be able to distinguish soldiers from humanitarian workers or aid activities from military action. It is worth recalling that USAID was originally established to separate military from nonmilitary aid.

It is also important to note that a significant amount of aid provided by the United States is frequently directed back to the United States or U.S. companies. Oftentimes, U.S. foreign aid agreements will contain requirements that certain items be procured from U.S. manufacturers or businesses. Many times U.S. consultants are hired under these grants and contracts. The end result is that a sizeable proportion of the aid dollars is channeled back to the donor country or entities within the donor country.

PRESIDENTIAL INITIATIVES

Presidential initiatives are another mechanism for targeted U.S. global health programs. There have been many presidential initiatives in the past decade but perhaps the most well-known of these is the President's Emergency Plan for AIDS Relief, also known by its acronym, PEPFAR. President George W. Bush announced this program during his January 2003 State of the Union Address as a five-year initiative to direct $15 billion to fifteen high-HIV-burden focus countries. PEPFAR was reauthorized in 2008 for an additional five years up to a total of $48 billion. The goals of PEPFAR are, quite simply, HIV prevention and treatment. Its activities include prevention of mother-to-child transmission of HIV, procuring antiretroviral drugs, and rolling out HIV treatment programs. Through PEPFAR support, some five million people have received HIV treatment with antiretrovirals, and more than forty-five million have received HIV counseling and testing. Approximately eleven million pregnant women were tested for HIV in 2012, which resulted in medications to prevent mother-to-child transmission dispensed to more than 750,000 HIV-infected pregnant women, which in turn led to about 250,000 infants being born HIV-free. [6] While there was initial discussion and disagreement about the most effective prevention methods (particularly when there was an earmark for abstinence-only teaching), there is general consensus among the international HIV control community that PEPFAR has resulted in tremendous progress in stemming the tide of HIV and has saved millions of lives.

THE WORLD BANK

Another important agency in global health is the World Bank. Established in 1944 as the International Bank for Reconstruction and Development, its original mission was to facilitate postwar reconstruction and development, which was done in conjunction with the Marshall Plan activities to rebuild Europe. The World Bank's present-day mandate is worldwide poverty alleviation, no small goal. It aims to accomplish this by investing in and empowering poor people to participate in their country's economic development and by creating a climate for investments, job development, and, consequently, sustainable economic growth. The World Bank is a major donor that provides funds directly to governments, either as direct aid or through loans. To some extent, World Bank support for specific health programs has been displaced by initiatives such as PEPFAR and grants from the Gates Foundation, but it is still supporting multicountry HIV control programs in collaboration with UNAIDS and other partners.

PHILANTHROPIC AND NONGOVERNMENTAL ORGANIZATIONS

Philanthropic organizations are also major stakeholders in global health. Many of these are large organizations well-known to us: the Rockefeller Foundation, the Ford Foundation, and the W. K. Kellogg Foundation. The Bill and Melinda Gates Foundation, established in 1994 on the premise that all lives, no matter where they are being led, have equal value, has brought philanthropic giving for global health to a new level. Their endowment is roughly $40 billion. Since they began, they have committed more than $30 billion in grants, and their 2013 grant payments alone totaled $3.6 billion. [7] These fund disbursements have been to different organizations and entities with a focus on scientific and technological breakthroughs that will result in exponential gains in global health. Under their global health programs, they have identified priority diseases or conditions to include TB, malaria, nutrition, diarrheal diseases, reproductive and maternal health, respiratory infections, and vaccine-preventable diseases such as polio.

As already mentioned, there are numerous nongovernmental organizations—both national and international—engaged in global health. These can be categorized in many ways, but one distinction is between organizations that are engaged in emergency relief versus those engaged in development. This distinction separates those that are on the front lines of the latest disaster, the first group on the ground establishing the portable medical units and dispensing emergency aid, the true first responders. These can be compared to the organizations that work with local groups and communities over time to develop sustainable practices and growth opportunities. Of course this distinction is not clear-cut. Many organizations associated with emergency relief, such as Médecins Sans Frontières/Doctors Without Borders, have both emergency response units and longer-term development projects focused on TB control (particularly multidrug-resistant TB) and have been present in several countries for years if not decades. Organizations that focus on long-term community building may find themselves in the position of providing emergency assistance when they happen to be in the epicenter of a sudden natural disaster. This was certainly the case with certain organizations following the 2004 tsunami in Asia and the 2010 earthquake in Haiti.

In the past, NGOs had the reputation of being small-scale players on the global health stage. This is certainly not true today. While there are many small organizations everywhere today, NGO and grassroots organizations are no longer synonymous with small-scale. Many of these organizations are implementing partners of large bilateral funders—receiving hundreds of millions of dollars from funders such as USAID—to execute large-scale multicountry programs or to serve as the lead of a consortium of NGOs. There are different ways one can evaluate both the efficiency and results of these organizations. Independent organizations such as GuideStar and the American Institute of Philanthropy Charity Rating Guide evaluate and rate the organization's efficiency, assess its overhead, and calculate how much of its budget is directed toward efforts in the field versus maintaining its headquarters staff. Anyone seeking to volunteer, to work, or to donate to one of these NGOs can now research important information on the organization's financial and organizational structure and see how it compares to its peers.

ACADEMIA AND RESEARCH

Lastly, in the cast of global health actors, we include academic and research institutions. This category includes influential, agenda-setting agencies in the United States such as the CDC or the National Institutes of Health, and also academic institutions including many U.S. medical schools and schools of public health. In many instances, it is the medical schools that are closely affiliated with their schools of public health or their international health departments that tend to play a larger role in global health. A visit to the websites of many medical and public health schools reveals how prevalent global health centers, institutes, and programs are at most of the schools with large research profiles. Many schools now have institutional partnerships and/or memoranda of understanding signed with at least one international collaborator. Fortunately, these partnerships have shifted from a former "colonial-style" relationship in which the U.S. institution drove the process, relied on host-country labor and patients, and reaped the sole benefits of academic recognition and publication. Today, equitable partnerships between institutions in the Global North are being formed with partners in the Global South; the multi-institutional U.S.–Kenya AMPATH consortium is one of the largest and oldest such relationships. [8]

CONCLUSION

This chapter is meant to provide a general overview and framework for thinking about the numerous stakeholders in global health. It is not meant to be an exhaustive list of all important agencies engaged in global health; any mention of specific organizations is intended for illustrative purposes only. As you delve deeper into the topic of global health, this chapter may provide you with a means to organize the different entities and how they relate to one another. One thing is clear: there are many organizations involved in global health—with a variety of roles, purposes, orientations—and a lot of overlap. Needless to say, coordination is a daunting task and is becoming more of a challenge as the number of stakeholders and players continues to increase.

REFERENCES

1. Lalremruata A, Ball M, Bianucci R, Welte B, Nerlich AG, Kun JF, et al. Molecular identification of falciparum malaria and human tuberculosis co-infections in mummies from the Fayum depression (Lower Egypt). *PLoS One.* 2013;8(4):e60307. doi: 10.1371/journal.pone.0060307. Epub 2013 Apr 2.

2. Preamble to the Constitution of the World Health Organization as adopted by the International Health Conference, New York, June 19–22, 1946; signed on July 22, 1946, by the representatives of sixty-one States (Official Records of the World Health Organization, no. 2, p. 100) and entered into force on 7 April 7, 1948. http://www.who.int/about/definition/en/print.html, accessed December 3, 2013.

3. U.S. Department of Health & Human Services website, About Us. http://www.hhs.gov/about/, accessed December 3, 2013.

4. USAID website. http://www.usaid.gov/what-we-do, accessed December 3, 2013.

5. International Rescue Committee website. http://www.rescue.org/news/aid-groups-urge-nato-separate-military-and-humanitarian-activities-protect-civilians-afghanista-4463, accessed December 3, 2013.

6. PEPFAR website, Latest Results. http://www.pepfar.gov/funding /results/, accessed on December 3, 2013.

7. Bill and Melinda Gates Foundation website, Foundation Fact Sheet. http://www.gatesfoundation.org/Who-We-Are/General-Information/ Foundation-Factsheet, accessed December 3, 2013.

8. AMPATH website. http://www.ampathkenya.org/, accessed December 3, 2013.

3

A BRIEF PRIMER
OF INFECTIOUS DISEASES

Humans, Their Environment, and Evolution

John R. Butterly

RELATIONSHIPS BETWEEN ORGANISMS

William Osler, who was considered the father of modern medicine, was quoted as saying that humanity has but three great enemies: fever, famine, and war. Of these, by far the greatest, by far the most terrible, is fever. What he meant by this was that he knew that even during famines and war, many more people died of infectious diseases—which cause fever—than they did from the direct effects of famine or wounds incurred in combat. While there was a point in the recent history of the developed nations where we thought we had conquered disease caused by infectious agents, we will learn in this chapter about the ability of microorganisms to adapt, and in chapter 11 we will learn how this trait enables pathogenic organisms to develop resistance to the antibiotics we develop to combat infectious disease. This will help us develop an understanding of why infectious diseases remain a major challenge to the health and well-being of our global society, whether we are resource-rich or resource-poor, whether we consider ourselves developed, developing, or underdeveloped. We will also explore the important biological connections we share with the very organisms we try so hard to either avoid or eradicate from our environment. The following is a brief introduction to our relationship with some of the organisms with which we share this planet, organisms that depend on us, in rather unpleasant ways, for their survival.

As biological entities, we share the earth with a number of fellow travelers. One of the characteristics of living organisms is that they have a strong tendency to develop mutual interdependence so that they live together, and frequently depend on one another, in specified ways. The biological term for this is "symbiosis," which essentially translates to "living together."

There are three basic forms of symbiosis:

- Parasitism, in which one organism benefits from the relationship but the other is harmed
- Commensalism, in which one organism benefits and the other is neither helped nor harmed (at least not measurably)
- Mutualism, in which both organisms benefit

We can use as an example of parasitism an insect called an ichneumon wasp. This small wasp, which is harmless to human beings, lays its eggs on other insects and tends to hide them either internally in a plant or in little mud dwellings that it creates. When the eggs hatch, the larvae burrow into the insect on which the egg has been laid and use the insect as a source of nutrition until it can pupate and develop into an adult wasp.

An example of commensalism might be the relationship between grazing cattle and different types of birds that are generically called "cattle birds" or cattle egrets. The birds feed on insects that the cattle disturb as they walk through their grazing territory; studies have shown that these birds can be three to four times as effective in their foraging when they associate with large grazing animals. [1] It is not clear whether the cattle benefits substantially or not (possibly by being warned of nearby predators) but the birds certainly do. In the plant world, epiphytic plants, such as orchids, benefit by living in the canopy of tropical rain forests. They grow on the tops of taller trees so they can benefit by being closer to sunlight, but they do not appear to benefit or harm the trees in any way.

Mutualism is the circumstance in which both organisms benefit. One example would be the relationship between butterflies and bees and the flowers from which they obtain nectar. The insects obviously benefit by gaining nutrition, but the plants also benefit by being pollinated by these insects. An excellent example of mutualism is given in an anecdote about Charles Darwin. He noticed that there was an orchid growing in Madagascar, the nectar of which was kept in an extremely long protuberance at the back of the flower. Darwin predicted that a moth would be discovered with a tongue that would be the same length as the protuberance in the flower, and twenty-one years after Darwin's death, this moth was discovered. It was found that this moth can only feed on this particular orchid and that the moth is the only animal able to pollinate the flower, thereby ensuring survival of both the moth and orchid. The most extreme example of mutualism is found in eukaryotic cells. Unlike prokaryotic cells, such as bacteria, eukaryotic cells have inclusions within the cellular body known as organelles. Of particular interest among these organelles are the mitochondria. The mitochondria are considered the power packs or energy boosters in the cell as it is here that aerobic respiration occurs. Mitochondria have their own DNA that does not mix with the nuclear DNA. It has been determined that mitochondria were at one point free-living organisms and developed a relationship of mutualism with other cells so that now mitochondria are no longer found as free-living organisms, and all eukaryotic cells now contain (and depend upon) mitochondria.

These relationships are of relevance to us as they describe the different interactions we have with the myriad of microorganisms that live on and in our bodies. All of us, from the moment of birth, become colonized with bacteria on our skin, on our mucous membranes, and in our bowels. Some of these colonizers develop commensal relationships with us, the hosts, while many, if not most, of these relationships are those of mutualism, as will be described shortly. In contrast to these beneficial interactions, infectious diseases are a specific form of parasitism, in which the parasite (in most cases a virus, a bacterium, or a single-celled eukaryotic parasite such as the plasmodia that cause malaria) is the agent that benefits, and the host (in this case, us) suffers harm.

We should start with definitions that will enable us to understand this process. We define infection as the establishment of a microorganism on or in a host. This may be a short-lived process, and the host is usually unaware of and may benefit from this relationship, as we noted above. This is specifically called colonization, and a good example of this would be the bacteria that live on our skin and in our large intestines. They generally do not cause infectious disease and in fact confer specific benefits by protecting us from colonization and subsequent infection by organisms that are not benign. On the other hand, an infectious disease is the establishment of a microorganism that does cause a disease that can damage the host. This generally is not an asymptomatic situation but will produce clinical signs and symptoms consistent with the specific disease. When an organism produces such an infectious process, we refer to it as a pathogen. Pathogens are microorganisms with the capacity to cause disease, that is, pathology. We can divide pathogens into a number of different types but for the purpose of this chapter, let's consider two basic types. *Principal pathogens* are those that cause disease in most organisms they infect. *Opportunistic pathogens,* on the other hand, only cause disease in organisms that have been weakened in some way. The degree of ability of a pathogenic organism to cause disease is referred to as *virulence.* Virulence is a word that comes from the Latin base *viru,* which means poison. The more virulent or poisonous an organism is, the stronger its ability to cause disease. The virulence of an organism is determined by host characteristics as well as by the pathogen's intrinsic characteristics.

There are a number of factors that determine how a microbe will interact with the host. Is the host likely to encounter the organism (determined by how prevalent the organism is in the environment, whether there are environmental protections such as safe drinking water and adequate sanitation, and whether the population in question is adequately immunized or otherwise immune due to prior exposure or other factors)? If the microorganism is encountered, can it gain entry into the host? If the microbe does gain entry, does it have the ability to grow within the host, and does it have the ability to avoid host defenses? Once the organism is growing within the host, does it have the ability to invade tissue, and might it have a particular predilection or tropism for particular tissue? (For example, rabies virus is very specific for tissue of nerves and the brain.) Once the organism has invaded the tissue, does the organism have the ability to reproduce and be transferred to another host?

The traits we are talking about are called *virulence factors,* gene products that increase the ability of a microorganism to cause disease. These can include toxins that directly cause symptoms such as vomiting, diarrhea, or, in the case of botulism, paralysis, or other specialized proteins that are produced to neutralize host defenses, evade tissue barriers, adhere to host tissues, or actually invade and destroy the host's tissues.

Considering the larger picture of infectious diseases, as we talk about pathogenic organisms that can cause specific diseases in specific hosts, we begin to understand that this relationship implies a degree of "relatedness" between the pathogen and the host. For example, the virus for the common cold is highly contagious for human beings and some other mammals, but other mammals such as dogs are completely unaffected by this virus and it does not have the capability to adhere to canine tissues or invade the canine body. On the other hand, the bowel parasite *Toxocara canis* is a specific parasite of canines. This organism causes the commonly found infection of dogs with bowel worms but cannot cause that infection in humans. Because it does not recognize cellular messages in human tissue, rather than finding its way through the circulation to the lungs and then to the GI tract, it will cause a self-limited disease known as *visceral larva migrans* in which the larva of this worm will wander throughout tissues in the human being and cause a self-limited febrile illness, but the larva eventually die without causing a sustained parasitic infection that can be transmitted to other hosts.

The characteristics of pathogens include the ability to breach defenses of the normal host including anatomic defenses such as the skin, cellular defenses such as the cellular immune system, and biochemical defenses that might be found in the blood of the host such as antibodies. Pathogens develop these traits through a genomic armamentarium of traits that are missing in nonpathogenic strains. We can characterize some of these traits as defensive traits or offensive traits. For example, the bacteria *Haemophilus influenzae* can create a protease (an enzyme that inactivates specific proteins) that will destroy a specific antibody known as immunoglobulin A. Immunoglobulin A is specifically found in the secretions of the respiratory tract and *Haemophilus influenzae* is a respiratory infectious agent. You can see where this would help defend the *Haemophilus influenzae* bacteria from being destroyed and allow it to establish itself in its host.

The organism that causes syphilis, known as *Treponema pallidum,* can coat itself with a human protein known as fibronectin so that it can hide from antibodies within human blood and therefore avoid being destroyed, kind of a cellular hermit crab. A third defensive mechanism would be that used by *Mycobacterium tuberculosis,* the organism that causes tuberculosis. This organism can stimulate the host to produce interleukin 10, which is a powerful immuno-suppressive agent or cytokine, which suppresses the host defenses so the bacteria can continue to grow. [2, 3]

HOW WE PROTECT OURSELVES

As we have often heard, the best defense is a good offense. Examples of offensive characteristics include the development of adhesions, invasins, or specific toxins that enable the organism to adhere to intestinal mucosa and thereby invade and cause dysentery and diarrhea. The organism that causes cholera produces a toxin known as cholera toxin that can bind to cells lining the intestine, known as enterocytes, which increases cyclic AMP, which subsequently inhibits sodium absorption and increases chloride secretion. The ultimate result of this is an extremely profuse, watery diarrhea (shedding millions of cholera bacteria into the environment) that can prove fatal if not immediately treated with fluid and electrolyte replacement. A third offensive characteristic would be contagion factors. A good example of this is the contagion factor of the common cold, which causes mucus discharge and sneezing, which can effectively spread the virus throughout the environment.

Genetically it has been shown that as bacteria evolve, they start as free-living organisms that can live in multiple habitats and can infect multiple hosts, but relatively ineffectually. Through the dual evolutionary processes of genetic mutation and natural selection, they can become extremely effective pathogens, but in doing so they become host restricted, which means they can only infect particular species and become obligate parasites that can no longer live freely in the environment and require a specific host to continue to live and be transmitted to other organisms. Another term used to describe this is endosymbionts, or organisms that require living within another organism, that is, obligate intracellular organisms. These specific pathogens become extremely success-ful virulent organisms that are generally highly contagious within their specific hosts, but are harmless to most other hosts.

As these organisms evolve, we see a genomic change in their genetic material. That is, an originally diverse, extensive genomic library undergoes a reduction in genomic size with an accumula-tion of inactive or defective genes, but it also accumulates special-ized genes that are specific virulence factors.

An excellent example of this specified evolution is found in the genus Bordetella. *Bordetella bronchosepticus* survives in the environ-ment in a facultative way, which means it can live in multiple envi-ronments both with and without oxygen, is able to infect multiple animal hosts, but is not very contagious, not easily transmitted to other hosts.

A closely related organism, *Bordetella pertussis,* is the organism that produces whooping cough in human beings. This organism cannot live free in the environment and is limited to humans as the only host, but for us it is extremely contagious and virulent. It is an obligate parasite but a very effective one. [4, 5]

When we classify pathogens, we classify them either as infec-tious agents such as viruses (smallpox being an example); prokary-otes, which are the bacteria such as streptococcus and staphylococ-cus; or as parasites that are generally eukaryotes, which are either unicellular or multicellular organisms. Examples of unicellular or-ganisms include protozoans such as the trypanosomes or plasmo-dium, the latter being the infectious agent of malaria. Multicellular organisms include certain metazoans such as the hookworm and other intestinal parasites.

ANCESTRAL DISEASES AND DISEASES
OF CIVILIZATION

We discussed earlier in this chapter how organisms that cause infection evolve along with their hosts so that they can become more effective in their ability to invade, multiply, and increase their transmission, although this is at the expense of limiting the diversity of hosts they are able to infect. This brings us to a discussion of the ancestral diseases versus the diseases of civilization: that is, those that developed along with us as we evolved from a common ancestor with other primates into hunter-gatherers living in an ancestral environment, as opposed to those that began to appear as we socially evolved through a pastoral to an agricultural environment.

The ancestral diseases tend to be endemic, which means they are always present in the environment although they do not necessarily infect multiple individuals at any one time. Because of this they are not dependent on a large population for transfer and they either have a natural reservoir in the environment or tend to be chronic diseases so they can be transmitted from individual to individual. These organisms cause diseases such as leprosy, yaws, malaria, and yellow fever.

Diseases of civilization, on the other hand, tend to be epidemic diseases; that is, they are not always present in large numbers at any one time in the environment, but as they encounter large numbers of susceptible individuals, they can infect large segments of the population. (This point will be important when we discuss vaccination and herd immunity.) These evolved from diseases that previously infected animals that were later domesticated by human beings (as we discussed in the genetic differences between *Bordetella bronchosepticus* and *Bordetella pertussis*). They require a herd effect; that is, they require large populations and some degree of prevalence in a society, as there is no natural reservoir. These diseases have evolved to become the major killers of humanity throughout history and include diseases such as smallpox, tuberculosis, measles, falciparum malaria (which evolved from an avian form of malaria, unlike the other forms of malaria which evolved in other primates), and influenza.

As we began to live more closely with animals, in either a semidomesticated or domesticated form, we increasingly became exposed to their pathogens. This can be seen in a pastoral culture, typified today by the Masai tribe who live in close contact with their cattle and drink a mixture of the cattle's milk and blood to satisfy their protein requirements, as well as in agricultural societies, where farmers live in close contact with their domestic livestock (at times in the same quarters), and even in our everyday life where we share our homes with our pets.

As we became exposed to the organisms associated with our domestic animals, and they to ours, we became increasingly likely to acquire the diseases they cause, and the organisms began to evolve to become progressively virulent human pathogens. Transfer of diseases from animals to humans can occur in a number of ways. For example, one can see incidental infections such as rabies in which humans are a dead-end host, that is, when a human being is infected, they usually do not infect any other individual and the virus is not passed on. An excellent example of an endemic infection that can be passed from animal to human beings is malaria, in which humans may be the only reservoir but transfer to another human being requires a vector, in this case a mosquito. Epidemic infections that can be passed from animals to humans are exemplified by the bubonic plague, which can be transmitted from rats to humans via the bite of a flea but can also be transferred from human to human via a respiratory process in cases of pneumonic plague. An important point to remember about an organism's ability to create epidemics is that if a pathogen acquires the ability to pass from human being to human being, and an animal vector is

no longer necessary, the pathogen can become extremely dangerous, as we saw in the SARS outbreak.

Examples of diseases and pathogens that have evolved from
an animal disease to a human disease include measles, which has
been shown to have evolved from the rinderpest virus of cattle;
tuberculosis, which seems to have evolved from a similar mycobacterium that infects cattle; the smallpox virus, which is directly
related to the cattle virus that causes cowpox; influenzae virus,
which evolved from viruses that infect swine and ducks; *Bordetella
pertussis*, which evolved from bacteria that causes more diffuse disease in multiple animals including pigs and dogs; and *falciparum malaria,* which originally evolved in birds such as chickens and ducks
before becoming a major pathogen in humans.

Another point to remember is that when humans and microbes
pathogenic to humans do not coexist over long periods of time,
the unexposed human population cannot develop a genetic memory of exposure to these organisms, and the results can be devastating. Examples of this include fatal epidemics of smallpox and measles that occurred in the indigenous populations of the Western
Hemisphere when these diseases were brought over by European
explorers.

The archeological literature has described evidence for rapid
and recent evolution of certain highly successful pathogens, including evidence of smallpox as early as 1600 BC and mumps in
400 BC. Examples from more contemporary times include polio,
first recognized in 1840; HIV/AIDS, which was first encountered in
1959 but not recognized until the 1980s; and Lyme disease, which
was first noted in 1962. The importance of the relatively recent
appearance of these pathogens, and the apparent accelerated evolution they seem to have undergone, will become obvious as we
discuss the development of antibiotic resistance and "super pathogens" in chapter 11.

How do we define success as defined by a pathogen? In general, we can define this by the ability to infect, to reproduce, and to transmit itself to other organisms. This can be through food or water such as salmonellosis and trichinosis, transmission by a vector such as seen in malaria or sleeping sickness, through contact with genital or skin lesions such as seen in syphilis and smallpox, coughing or sneezing as seen with the common cold, or transmission via diarrhea and fecal/oral spread or contamination of the water supply such as we see with cholera and polio.

Success as defined by the host is related to the evolution of genetic defense mechanisms. These can protect populations against diseases that are endemic in their environment, either by conferring immunity or, most often, by mitigating the effects of the diseases caused by these pathogens. There are a number of genetic traits such as sickle cell disease, thalassemia, and glucose-6 phosphate dehydrogenase deficiency, all of which cause certain amounts of anemia when present as a single gene or heterozygous state, but also confer relative protection against severe malarial infection in the populations living in endemic areas. Other diseases such as Tay-Sachs disease, found in people of Ashkenazi Jewish background, may protect against severe tuberculosis infection. The genetic defect that causes cystic fibrosis, also found in people of European descent, may protect against typhoid fever when present in the heterozygous state, and the genetic defect that causes phenylketonuria may protect against fetal miscarriage caused by mycotoxins found in certain diets when found in the heterozygous state.

When we wonder why these heterozygous states persist in the population even though the homozygous state of these defects is often fatal before the individual is able to reproduce, we begin to understand that it is because the heterozygous state actually advantages the individual with the single defective gene. Because of this, the gene pool of that particular population is able to develop what is called a balanced polymorphism, which means that the presence of this defective gene will persist in a ratio in a population that is determined by the prevalence of the disease against which it protects, and the relative degree of protection it confers upon the individual carrying that gene—that is, if it confers enough advantage so that the individual can reproduce and pass the defective gene on to his or her descendants, the gene will persist in that gene pool.

SUMMARY

To reiterate important points made in the preceding pages, an infectious process, which may or may not cause harm, depends on a complex interaction between the pathogen's and the host's characteristics. The interaction between the pathogen and host implies, in fact requires, a substantial degree of relatedness between the infecting organism and the host. Finally, we have learned that the diseases of humanity that are of significance have evolved with us, and their relative pathogenicity is in large part determined by us.

As we learn about epidemiological principles in the following chapter, the recrudescence of infectious diseases in what we refer to as the developed world, and the continuous emergence of pathogenic organisms resistant to even the most significant antibiotics, we can begin to understand that this interrelatedness of living organisms will play a major role in the ongoing struggle between the evolutionary ability of organisms to genetically enhance their effectiveness as pathogens and our technological ability to defeat them and cure the diseases they cause.

REFERENCES

1. Grubb, T. Adaptiveness of foraging in the cattle egret. *Wilson Bulletin,* 1976. 88 (1): 145–48.

2. Hornef MW, Wick MJ, Rhen M, Normark S. Bacterial strategies for overcoming host innate and adaptive immune responses. *Nat Immunol.* 2002; 3: 1033–40.

3. Mandell GL, Bennett JE, Dolin R. Principles & practice of infectious diseases. 6th ed. Philadelphia: Elsevier, 2010.

4. Parkhill J, Sebaihia M, Preston A et al. Comparative analysis of the genome sequence of Bordetella pertussis, Bordetella parapertussis, and Bordetella bronchoseptica. *Nat Genet.* 2003; 35: 32–40.

5. Finley BB, Falkow S. Common themes in microbial pathogenicity revisited. *Microbio Mol Biol Rev.* 1997; 61: 136–69.

4

EPIDEMIOLOGY AND INFECTIOUS DISEASES

Introduction and Early Perspectives

John R. Butterly

A PERPLEXING CASE

In 1978, a patient with an unusual presentation was admitted to a major urban hospital. The patient was a thirty-eight-year-old gay urologist admitted with a history of five days of fever. He was brought to the emergency room by his significant other, and at that time he was hypoxic, which means he had a low oxygen content in his blood, and he was poorly responsive. His white blood cell count was low, only 3,000, which was unusual since people who have infections generally have high white blood cell counts. Despite all efforts, including multiple antibiotics, vasoactive agents given intravenously to raise his dangerously low blood pressure, intubation, and mechanical ventilation, he died of cardiovascular collapse eight hours after admission. This patient sticks in my mind because we had no idea why he died, or from what he died. We will return to this case at the end this section.

EPIDEMIOLOGY: INTRODUCTION AND DEFINITIONS

Epidemiology is defined as the study of health-related events in defined populations. It is called that because the science was originally the study of epidemics. There are a number of terms in the science of epidemiology, and it is important to understand their specific meaning since much of the global health literature incorporates these terms in the text. The word *endemic* comes from the Greek *endemos,* or dwelling in a place. It is used to describe a disease or pathogen that is present or usually prevalent in a population or geographical area. The word *epidemic* comes from the Greek *epideios,* which means prevalent, and describes a level of disease prevalence that occurs suddenly and in numbers clearly in excess of normal expectancy. *Pandemic* comes from the Greek root *pan,* which means all, and *demos,* which means people. This word is used to describe widespread epidemics that involve multiple regions or at times the entire globe.

Other important definitions include *incidence,* which is the rate of occurrence of new cases of infection or diseased patients per unit of population per time. This can be considered the inflow of diseased individuals to the existing population. The word *prevalence,* on the other hand, refers to the number of current cases of diseased individuals in the population per unit of time. It is important to note that *this is not a rate* but a snapshot picture at any point. Cure of a disease or mortality or death from the disease is considered the outflow of diseased individuals that affect the prevalence of the disease.

While changes in incidence, cure, or mortality (all of which are rates) can usually be considered to be good or bad trends depending on whether they are going up or down (for example, increasing cure can always be considered as good), the same cannot be said of prevalence (which is not a rate). Consider a tub of water with a faucet or inflow representing the incidence of cases, which is the number of cases per unit of population per time. Outflow, which is the cure rate of the disease or the mortality, would be the tub's drain. The amount of water in the tub at any one time, which would depend on the rate of water flowing in vs. the rate of water draining out, would be the prevalence, or the number of cases per unit of population at any one time (but not per unit time).

What happens to prevalence if we prolong survival by decreasing mortality? In this case, the level of water in the tub would increase to the point at which the outflow mortality rate again balances with the inflow or incidence. In this scenario, prevalence of the disease has increased. While we have not cured the disease, we have prolonged survival, and the increased prevalence is a good thing. On the other hand, what if we do increase the cure rate; what happens to the prevalence then? Prevalence then will decrease until the outflow or cure rate is again equal to the inflow or incidence of the disease. In this instance, prevalence has markedly decreased, this time due to an actual cure of the disease, and the decrease in prevalence is also a good thing because fewer people are dying (and also more people are living longer, as they did when we prolonged survival without cure). We can see, however, that increasing mortality would decrease the prevalence the same as increasing cure. If we decrease prevalence by increasing mortality, it actually is a bad outcome, so in this case a decrease in prevalence is undesirable. While this may seem confusing at first, it is important to recognize these relationships because the tendency is to think that increased prevalence is always bad and decreased prevalence is always good. As you can see, it depends on the total relationship between the rate of incidence of the disease and the rate of mortality or cure.

THE BEGINNINGS OF MODERN EPIDEMIOLOGY

The history of epidemiology begins with a gentleman by the name of John Snow. In 1849, Snow published a pamphlet called "On the Mode of Communication of Cholera" in which he proposed that the "cholera poison" (no one at the time knew about the bacterial cause of disease or bacterial toxins) reproduced in the human body and was spread through the contamination of water. This theory was opposed to the more commonly accepted idea that cholera, as was thought about many diseases at the time, was transmitted through the inhalation of foul air. Because there was no technology Snow could use to prove his theory, his concept did not gain acceptance. At the time, London was supplied by two water companies. One of the companies took its water out of the Thames River upstream of the main city while the second obtained its water downstream from the city (and from sewage outflow from the streets of London). It wasn't until 1854, when, during a second cholera epidemic in London, Snow did a study in which he put points on a map of the area involved and was able to determine that the majority of cases of cholera clustered around one public pump where people got their fresh water. Higher concentration of cholera was noted around the pump on Broad Street, which obtained water contaminated by the city's sewage. With some difficulty, Snow was able to talk the Public Health Board into removing the handle of the Broad Street pump that supplied water to this neighborhood, and the epidemic was contained. Once this was done, the incidence of cholera quickly decreased. Because of this first epidemiological study, Snow is considered the father of modern epidemiology.

At the same time, Florence Nightingale, who is also recognized as a leader in epidemiologic studies and disease, made highly significant contributions. During the Crimean War, Nightingale, against the advice of her family, went to Crimea to help soldiers wounded in battle. It became clear to her that the vast majority of deaths in the army in the Crimea were due to preventable disease and a small fraction were from wounds (remember the quote from Osler). In tracking the causes of death she was able to show that this was due to the horrible, filthy conditions under which the wounded were hospitalized. She and her group of nurses began a process of cleaning the hospital and equipment and reorganizing patient care. At the time, ten times as many soldiers died from illnesses such as typhus, typhoid, cholera, and dysentery than died from battle wounds. Nightingale reported these conditions on the health of the army to the Royal Commission (it helped that her family was friends of the minister of health at the time). Resources were put in to improve these conditions, and her efforts were rewarded by substantial decreases in mortality rates.

EARLY THEORIES OF DISEASE

While it seems obvious to us now, the reason Johns Snow's and Florence Nightingale's actions were so innovative at the time is because no one had any idea what caused these diseases. (Prior to the modern era when people referred to disease, they were really talking about infectious diseases as opposed to the chronic, metabolic diseases such as hypertension, diabetes, and coronary disease that now affect the populations of developed nations.) At the time, and for centuries prior, the theories of disease included the theories of divine retribution, an imbalance of "humors" in the body, and the miasma theory.

The theory of divine retribution held that if somebody developed an illness such as smallpox or the bubonic plague, it was because they were bad people or had done something evil, and the illness was visited upon them as divine retribution. While this may have been a convenient theory from the perspective of those who were not ill (who were almost always more well-off and living in more sanitary conditions than those who suffered in greater numbers), in the present day it is considered bad form to blame a patient for his or her illness! Another working theory was that diseases were caused by an imbalance of "humors" or fluids within the body for example the balance between things such as blood and bile. It was this concept that led to such medical therapies as bleeding individuals who were ill, taking their blood by the application of leeches, or placing burning paper on their skin to raise blisters and draw out the bad humors. It is not difficult to understand why people might have feared physicians. Finally, there was the theory of miasma, which held that a disease was carried in contaminated air. One assumes that this was because one found large concentrations of disease in areas of open sewage or contamination, and the foul air associated with that was felt to carry the disease. The obvious example of this is malaria, the name of which comes from the Italian *mal,* or bad, and *aria,* which means air; it was felt to be the miasma or bad air around swamps that carried malaria, although of course we know now that the disease is carried by the mosquitoes that breed in the swamp.

We learned in the previous chapter about our relationship with the organisms that cause infectious diseases, how they developed pathogenic or virulent traits, and how we might have developed defenses against them. How did we finally come to understand how these diseases were caused and transmitted? In the early eighteenth century, optical experimentation was just beginning. A fellow named Anton van Leeuwenhoek began to experiment with lenses that enabled him to develop an instrument that substantially improved microscopic powers. This was a hobby of his as he made his living as a drapery merchant. When Leeuwenhoek took some water from a pond and put it under his microscope, he discovered much to his surprise living microscopic organisms, which he referred to as animalcules. He noted that these were beautiful organisms with substantial internal structure; most importantly he noted that they were alive. Here was an entire universe of living organisms that had hitherto been unsuspected.

The importance of this, however, did not become apparent until almost two hundred years later, in the latter portion of the nineteenth century. At that time Louis Pasteur was doing his first work as a consultant to a brewery firm on the science of fermentation and pasteurization. It was by this work that he discovered that there were microscopic organisms, in the case of fermentation yeasts, that enabled solutions of sugar to be fermented to alcoholic beverages, and that there were also organisms that if allowed to contaminate the brew, would spoil the process by turning the alcohol to vinegar. During his experimentation with what we call pasteurization, which is rapid heating and cooling of liquids or food, he was able to determine that the spoilage of these products was due to bacteria. It was that work that eventually led to other discoveries, including the development of the vaccine for rabies.

At the time, because rabies is caused by a virus (remember the Latin root *viru* means poison), no infectious agent that was causing this disease could be identified under a microscope. His inability to view the agent together with the fact that the agent passed through filters that would remove all microscopic organisms then known to man, Pasteur felt that the causative agent was a toxin or poison, and he named it a virus. Using previous work with vaccinations by Edward Jenner (as we will talk more about later in this book), Pasteur was able to develop an effective vaccine that saved the life of a young child who had been bitten by a rabid animal. This was remarkable as no human being previously exposed to rabies in that way had ever survived. It is noteworthy that although Pasteur developed the vaccine, because he was not a physician he had to ask a physician friend to administer the vaccine.

The final chapter in this story involves a man named Robert Koch, who finally proved the causative relationship between disease and a microorganism, in this case the disease anthrax and its associated bacillus. He developed a series of postulates, known as Koch's postulates, that are as follows:

1. In order to prove that an organism is causative of a particular disease, the organism in question must be found in all animals with the disease but not in healthy animals. Koch recognized that there was such a thing as a carrier state, in which case an animal could be carrying the organism with no manifestation of the disease.

2. The organism must be isolated from a diseased animal and then grown in pure culture.
3. The organism causes the disease when introduced in a healthy animal.
4. The organism must then be re-isolated from the experimentally infected animal.

The third postulate introduces prohibitive ethical issues involving human disease and clinical experimentation, which have not always been acknowledged historically. Dr. Koch was awarded the Nobel Prize in 1905 for work demonstrating the causal relationship between microbes and tuberculosis.

THE DYNAMICS OF DISEASE TRANSMISSION

Today we take the germ theory of disease for granted, but we have only really understood this concept for slightly more than a hundred years. Now that we know about germs (the general term we use for bacteria, viruses, and at times parasites), we can think about how these agents are transmitted, and from there begin to understand how we might decrease the incidence of disease (and therefore the prevalence, morbidity, and mortality).

Infectious agents can be transmitted in a number of ways. A common means of disease transmission is through contaminated food or water. The food or water might be contaminated by a food preparer who has not washed his or her hands, or a water supply might be contaminated by contact with sewage. Another mode of transmission is by *fomites,* which refers to physical structures within the environment such as furniture or doorknobs. Vectors are common transmitters of disease. These can be mechanical vectors (such as a housefly that lands on an infected substance such as feces and then flies to a food source) or biological vectors, the most widely known example of which is the Anopheles mosquito that transmits the parasite that causes malaria. Finally, diseases can be airborne. By this we do not mean droplets or mists that are generated when someone sneezes, but pathogens that are suspended in the air such as tuberculosis or aerosols as one would see in the smog of heavily polluted air. A common example of a disease with airborne transmission is measles, which due to vaccination is not presently seen in developed nations. This fact becomes an obvious concern as one thinks about the possibilities of bioterrorism and weaponization of diseases such as anthrax or smallpox.

ANALYZING DATA: TESTING OUR HYPOTHESES THROUGH SCIENTIFIC STUDY

We are able to add to our knowledge of diseases by doing epidemiologic analysis of how, where, and when these diseases occur. These studies that help us to describe the patterns of disease occurrence identify the outbreaks, facilitate the identification of infectious agents, describe the occurrence of an asymptomatic infection if it occurs, and assist the understanding of pathogenesis, or the way in which the agent causes disease. These studies also allow us to identify and characterize the chain of infection, develop and evaluate treatment protocols, develop and evaluate primary, secondary, and tertiary preventive controlled measures in individuals, and describe and assess community-wide preventive measures.

Within epidemiologic studies, the gold standard is the clinical trial, specifically the randomized, placebo-controlled, double-blind clinical trial. These trials can be descriptive, analytical, observational, or experimental. A descriptive study would describe the existing distribution of case characteristics without regard to causal or other hypotheses, for example, a surveillance of toxigenic E. coli infections within a population. An analytical study would be designed to examine associations, particularly hypothesized causal relationships such as case control, cohort clinical trials, or cross-sectional surveys. An example of this would be the Framingham study that longitudinally followed the population of Framingham, Massachusetts, in trying to determine causal relationships between problems such as hypertension, diabetes, elevated cholesterol, and death from heart disease. Observational studies make up the bulk of epidemiologic research and focus on events, exposures, and diseases that occur in the population during the course of a normal life. Experimental studies, on the other hand, study the conditions under the direct control of the investigator.

Studies that involve human experimentation must be conducted with the oversight of an institutional review board (IRB) or human subjects committee (HSC). This was not always the case. The institution of these review boards came directly from the outcomes of the Nuremberg trials after World War II in which Nazi physicians in the concentration camps were held accountable for the human experimentation on prisoners without their consent.

Although these particular experiments were particularly horrific and had no real scientific basis behind them, experiments on human beings without their consent have also occurred in the United States. In the Tuskegee syphilis study carried out between 1932 and 1972 by the U.S. Public Health Service, poor sharecroppers in Tuskegee, Alabama (universally poor and black), who were known to have syphilis were studied to determine the natural history of the disease without being offered any treatment whatsoever, even after a cure became available. This was obviously unethical in addition to being racist. In 1956, at an institution on Staten Island, New York, known as Willowbrook, children who were institutionalized because of special needs were purposefully exposed to hepatitis A virus, both in the form of contaminated water, food, and capsules containing feces from individuals with the disease, so that the transmission of the disease could be studied. While this satisfied Koch's postulates (remember our earlier caveat on the third postulate), it clearly failed to satisfy even the most basic ethical principles as we would understand them today.

Even the most ethical and carefully composed clinical trial may lead to misleading results if it is not established with the proper design and statistical power. Mark Twain popularized the saying, "There are three kind of lies: lies, damned lies, and statistics." The first person who actually said this is not really known, but Twain ascribed it to Benjamin Disraeli. In 1988 a well-done, multicenter, randomized, double-blind, placebo-controlled trial of more than 17,000 patients called ISIS-2 (International Study of Infarct Survival) was published in the medical journal *The Lancet*. This study was done on patients admitted to the hospital with heart attacks (treated with either the clot-busting agent streptokinase, aspirin, or both). Findings were remarkable and incontrovertible in that there was a highly statistically significant benefit for both treatments either separately or, more importantly, given together. When they were given together, the effect was synergistic. That is, the benefit was greater than the arithmetic sum of either one separately. The statisticians of this study were particularly sophisticated and offered to demonstrate that even in a study this well done and with this many patients, if you tried to answer questions the study had not been designed to answer, you could come up with incorrect (and in this setting patently absurd) answers. In order to do this, the statisticians did a subgroup analysis evaluating the effects analyzed by astrological sign. What they found was that although the synergistic beneficial effect for streptokinase and aspirin was clearly present in people born into the sign of Gemini, there was no such benefit for individuals born under the sign of Libra. This effect was also statistically significant (although not to a p value less than 0.00001).

INFECTIOUS DISEASE IN THE UNITED STATES

The medical leadership of the United States decided it was time to close the book on infectious disease by the 1960s, as it was felt that the major infectious diseases had been conquered. They were either diseases of infrastructure that were solved through public health measures of clean drinking water and effective sewage treatment, for example cholera, typhus, and typhoid, or they were diseases amenable to vaccination such as smallpox and polio. But it was a premature announcement. About 10 years later, the National Academy of Sciences Institute of Medicine reported on social, political, and economic factors that led to a resurgence of infectious disease in the United States. These factors included microbial adaptation; human susceptibility; a change in climate and weather; changes in the ecosystem; human demographics and behavior; economic development and land use; international travel and commerce, technology, and industry; a breakdown of public health measures; poverty; war and famine; and a lack of political will. In other words, pretty much everything. As we learned in the introduction to infectious diseases, pathogens are extremely adaptable, and their "will to survive," that is, their genetic ability to adapt to adversity, is every bit as strong as ours. It is doubtful that we will ever be able to relax our vigilance in protecting ourselves from these organisms. We will discuss this in more detail in chapter 11 on antibiotic resistance.

EPIDEMIOLOGY IN ACTION:
A PERPLEXING CASE DEMYSTIFIED

Let's go back now to the case originally presented. If you remember, this was a thirty-eight-year-old gay urologist admitted with a five-day febrile illness. He was hypoxic and poorly responsive on admission and had a low white blood cell count instead of a high one. His chest X-ray showed what we call a whiteout, where the lung spaces are all filled with fluid and therefore show a relatively dense and patchy whiteout consistent with diffuse pneumonia. Despite the best of efforts, the gentleman became progressively hypoxic even though he had a tube in his throat and was on mechanical ventilation on 100 percent oxygen. He died of cardiovascular collapse eight hours after admission. No one had any idea what was wrong with this gentleman or why he died. It appeared to be a severe but treatable pneumonia.

Three years later, in July of 1981, an article in the *New York Times* described a rare cancer, known as Kaposi's Sarcoma, that was seen in forty-one homosexual men. Doctors in New York and California had noticed that young men being seen in their emergency rooms were presenting with a rare form of rapidly fatal cancer, and the incidence of this was enough to call attention to and be reported in the literature. At the same time, emergency room doctors in New York City and San Francisco were seeing a lot of cases of an unusual type of pneumonia caused by *Pneumocystis carinii,* a relatively benign organism not known to cause pneumonia in otherwise healthy individuals. These patients were similar, if not identical, to our patient. One year later epidemiologists at the Centers for Disease Control and Prevention (CDC) found that these patients all had deficient immune systems and linked the illness to blood, coining the term acquired immune deficiency syndrome, or AIDS. This, of course, was only descriptive as the positive agent had yet to be identified.

For reasons that were not yet understood, the disease seemed to affect only certain groups. The initial causes that were considered were a cytomegalovirus infection, which was common in gay men, possibly the chronic use of amyl nitrite, popular for the enhancement of sexual experience, or immune overload from multiple infections. It was not known if this was contagious or if so how it was spread, but it was felt not to affect women; most, if not all, of the cases occurred in gay men. However, by 1981 it was known to be affecting IV drug users, and it was also recognized to have an increased incidence in Haitians (at the time Haiti was a common destination for sex tourism) and hemophiliacs (who require frequent transfusions of blood and blood products). Hence, the association with "the 4 H's": homosexuality, heroin, Haitians, and hemophiliacs.

In 1984, the Pasteur Institute in France isolated what is now known as HIV or human immunodeficiency virus, and in 1985 Robert Gallo confirmed, using modified Koch's postulates, that HIV was the causative agent of AIDS. (HIV/AIDS in the world today is covered in chapter 7.) We should keep in mind that this disease, which at first was rapidly and uniformly fatal, is now a disease we have controlled in developed nations (and have the wherewithal to control worldwide). This would not have been possible without the early work done by epidemiologists.

SUMMARY

The earliest work in determining the source of epidemics began even before there was accurate knowledge as to the cause of the underlying disease, as evidenced by the pioneering work of John Snow and Florence Nightingale, among others. The modern plagues of HIV/AIDS and MDR TB (multi-drug resistant tuberculosis) are more contemporary lessons in the importance of the science of epidemiology in the world of global health, but if that were not enough, we are reminded daily of the threat of potential health risks in the form of food contaminated with salmonella or enterotoxic E. coli, evolution of dangerous forms of H1N1 influenza, or novel zoonotic viral agents such as SARS-COV and MERS-cov. We depend on the ongoing vigilance and surveillance by epidemiologists and continued cooperation by all nations to enable us to contain, control, and hopefully eradicate these threats long before they become widespread.

5

EPIDEMIOLOGY OF INFECTIOUS DISEASES

Global Perspective

Lisa V. Adams

Infectious disease, which antedated the emergence of humankind, will last as long as humanity itself, and will surely remain, as it has been hitherto, one of the fundamental parameters and determinants of human history.

—William H. McNeill, *Plagues and Peoples* [1]

Wherever there is a critical density of human life, infectious disease will be a major factor in impacting the health and well-being of that population. This has been shown throughout time immemorial. Outbreaks of emerging diseases occurring every decade or so remind us that we are still in a war with microbial agents, hoping at best to stave off the next invasion for as long as possible.

DISEASE ERADICATION, ELIMINATION, AND CONTROL

To discuss the epidemiology of infectious diseases from a global perspective, certain terms should be defined. In the previous chapter, key epidemiologic terms such as incidence and prevalence were discussed. On a global scale, we will consider the language of addressing certain pandemics by defining the terms eradication, elimination, and control.

Quite simply, eradication is to render a disease extinct. A disease has been eradicated when, as the result of deliberate efforts, there is a permanent reduction to zero of the worldwide incidence of infection caused by a specific agent. Therefore, because this disease does not exist anywhere in the natural environment, intervention measures are no longer needed to prevent transmission. Smallpox is only disease that has been eradicated in our lifetime.

SIDEBAR 5-1

Today, smallpox is the only major human disease that has been eradicated, and it is worthwhile to compare smallpox and malaria and consider the differing traits of the pathogens and the diseases they cause to understand why we have been able to eradicate one but not yet the other. In both smallpox and malaria, there is no animal reservoir for either variola, the virus of smallpox, or the plasmodium that causes falciparum malaria, so only humans can be affected by either the virus or the plasmodium. On the other hand, once a person has been infected by the smallpox virus, there is lifelong immunity, but this is not true with malaria, as we discussed earlier. In smallpox, subclinical cases are rare and an infected person can be identified and isolated before transmitting the disease to somebody else, but subclinical cases of malaria are frequent and undetectable, for example in someone with acquired partial immunity. Therefore, somebody with malaria can easily move around in society and be bitten by multiple mosquitoes, which can then transmit the disease to other humans. In smallpox, infectivity or contagiousness does not precede overt symptoms, but this is not true of malaria. There is only one serotype of the

(continued)

SIDEBAR 5-1 (CONT.)

variola virus, so a vaccine was developed that could be effective against all virus strains, but this is not true of malaria, so no effective vaccine has yet been developed. In addition, the smallpox vaccine is very effective, and of course there is no effective vaccine against malaria. Finally, from a global political standpoint, there was a major commitment by the World Health Organization and governments to eradicate smallpox, but this remains an open question in regards to malaria. Considering these points, compare smallpox to polio as well to help understand why the eradication of polio will also prove more difficult than the eradication of smallpox.

Elimination of a disease is achieved when, as the result of deliberate efforts, there is a reduction to zero of the incidence of infection in a defined geographical area. In this case, however, continued measures to prevent re-establishment of transmission of the disease *are* required. Two examples of diseases that we have eradicated in the United States are measles and polio. Though we no longer see indigenous cases of these diseases in the United States, outbreaks in other countries remind us we still need to keep our guard up. For example, to prevent the re-establishment of transmission of these diseases locally, childhood vaccination against measles and polio is still recommended in the United States.

Control is the last term to define. A disease has been controlled when, as the result of deliberate efforts, the reduction of disease incidence, prevalence, morbidity or mortality is at a locally acceptable level. In this case, continued intervention measures are required to maintain that reduction. There are several examples of diseases that are under control, or for which efforts to control them are underway, such as diarrheal diseases, tuberculosis, and HIV. Control of a disease is the first line of defense and consequently, national tuberculosis control and HIV control programs exist in most countries.

DISEASE SURVEILLANCE

To determine if our control, elimination, or eradication efforts are being effective, data need to be carefully collected, which is accomplished through disease surveillance. Surveillance can be defined as the ongoing, systematic collection, analysis, and interpretation of health-related data. Each of these steps is essential to the process. The data selected for surveillance purposes ought to be critical to the planning, implementation, and evaluation of the specific public health program or activity. It is also important to disseminate the results and data interpretation in a timely manner to a few important audiences. First and foremost, data should go to those responsible for program implementation, and particularly those responsible for collecting the data. Seeing the impact the data can have goes a long way toward improving data quality. Secondly, data should be shared with those in a position to make decisions about public health programming and resource allocation. This allows evidence-based policymaking. In addition to assessing the status of a particular disease or public health program, surveillance data can also be used to define public health priorities and to stimulate research to address gaps identified in the care and/or control of a disease.

In the United States, disease surveillance is conducted by local and national health authorities—city, county, and state health departments—that collect data on certain defined diseases which are reported up the chain from city to county to state and then eventually to the U.S. Centers for Disease Control and Prevention (CDC) in Atlanta. In other countries, disease surveillance is done by the district or regional health offices, and, in a similar fashion, they report their data upstream to a unit within their ministry of health. On the global level, the World Health Organization (who) is the final receiving entity for all global disease surveillance data. This affords the who officials the ability to evaluate disease control efforts and, by viewing the big picture of standardized disease reporting, to detect new disease outbreaks early. By mapping global surveillance data, the who can distinguish a spurious spike of cases in one country from an emerging regional outbreak. To ensure complete reporting, member states of the who are legally required to report certain diseases of public health significance, including yellow fever, plague, and cholera. There are a few other entities involved in global disease surveillance, such as the u.s. Department of Defense, which has a global emerging infections network. This is logical when one considers the potential of disease outbreaks to impact any of the department's operations and also the importance of identifying possible acts of bioterrorism.

The impact of a disease on a person or a population can be measured most simply in terms of morbidity and mortality. Mortality is a measure of deaths attributed to a particular disease, while morbidity is the impact that a disease has on your well-being. A group of diseases that cause significant morbidity, but not necessarily mortality, is the neglected tropical diseases. Collectively, these diseases are estimated to affect about one-sixth of the world's population, more than a billion people. Fortunately, effective and inexpensive (and now in most cases donated) treatment exists for these diseases. Tragically, treatment was reaching too few of those affected, hence their name of "neglected tropical diseases." Many of these diseases had been under the radar of global public health priorities because they were not directly causing deaths. A better understanding of the disabilities caused by some of these diseases, however, reveals how they do contribute to premature mortality. But even without death as a direct outcome, these diseases can profoundly affect an individual's functioning, which often impacts that person's livelihood as well as his or her family and community.

LIST OF THE SEVENTEEN NEGLECTED TROPICAL DISEASES

- Buruli ulcer (*Mycobacterium ulcerans* infection)
- Chagas disease
- Dengue/Severe dengue
- Dracunculiasis (guinea-worm disease)
- Echinococcosis
- Foodborne trematodiases
- Human African trypanosomiasis (sleeping sickness)
- Leishmaniasis
- Leprosy
- Lymphatic filariasis
- Onchocerciasis (river blindness)
- Rabies
- Schistosomiasis
- Soil-transmitted helminthiases
- Taeniasis/Cysticercosis
- Trachoma
- Yaws (endemic treponematoses)

THE CASE OF GUINEA WORM

Guinea worm is an excellent example of a neglected tropical disease that, due to a coordinated, well-funded, and creative international effort, is on the verge of eradication. The Latin name of the organism responsible for this scourge is *Dracunculus medinensis,* which loosely translates to "affliction with dragons." The appropriateness of this name will quickly become apparent. In some African countries, this disease is called the "empty granary" disease because this condition is so debilitating that it causes farmers to let their fields lay fallow and eventually their granaries empty. Guinea worm is an ancient disease; there is evidence of infection in the remains of the early Egyptians, and some scholars have questioned whether the Old Testament description of the fiery serpent that tortured the Israelites in the desert is a literary reference to guinea worm.

Guinea worm, a roundworm parasite, affected about fifty million people across northwest and central Africa, southwest Asia, the West Indies, and South America during the nineteenth and twentieth centuries. Due to its relation to the presence of surface water, it has a seasonal variation. Important features of this disease that impact efforts to eradicate it are guinea worm has no animal host; there is no vaccine to prevent guinea worm; there is no curative treatment; and affected individuals do not acquire immunity after having this disease, therefore, repeated infections can occur.

In parasitology, understanding the organism's life cycle is the first step to understanding the disease pathogenesis and points at which one can intervene to disrupt its life cycle and thereby interrupt the process of further disease transmission. Infection is acquired by drinking fresh water that has been contaminated with cyclops water fleas carrying the guinea worm larvae. The water fleas die in the person's stomach, allowing the guinea worm larvae to penetrate the digestive tract wall. Outside of the gastrointestinal tract, they lodge into organ tissues, where they mature into adult forms over the next ten to twelve weeks. As they mature, they grow in length with the adult female worm reaching 50 to 120 cm in length with a diameter of about 1 mm; the adult male is only half that size. About a year later, the now pregnant female migrates to the subcutaneous or superficial tissues in the arms or legs, where she will cause a blistering ulcer to form. This allows her to eject her tail and discharge her larvae. Since the blister burns, the infected person wants to put the limb in cooling water. This allows the larvae to be released into a water source, where they can then be picked up by the cyclops, develop into the infective form during the next two to three weeks, and repeat the cycle

The blister an infected individual develops can be disfiguring as well as painful. In fact, the blister is so painful it often makes it impossible for the person to continue working or carrying out his or her normal tasks of daily living. When the blister ulcerates, it can also become secondarily infected, especially in settings where maintaining hygiene is a challenge. Secondary infections can lead to skin infections and abscesses.

Unfortunately, treatment of guinea worm infection is a slow and painful process. The adult worm can only be extracted slowly by pulling it out a few centimeters each day. If pulled too briskly, the worm will break, and there is no way to complete extraction. Secondary infection is very likely. Surgical excisions have been attempted, but they have not been found to be more effective than the slow, meticulous process of removal. It typically takes four weeks to extract a single worm. Prevention of guinea worm is critical. Efforts have focused on protecting sources of drinking water from becoming contaminated with the cyclops fleas and the guinea worm larvae. These efforts have coalesced under the international campaign to eradicate guinea worm.

GUINEA WORM ERADICATION

Well-coordinated and concerted efforts involving a myriad of partners have placed guinea worm eradication within reach. The leading program has been the Inch-by-Inch Program, a name that refers to both the treatment of guinea worm and the targeted efforts to eradicate it. The Inch-by-Inch Guinea Worm Eradication Program began in 1986, led by the Carter Center and involving the CDC and the WHO as key partners. This collaboration has assisted twenty countries in implementing national guinea worm eradication programs. A primary intervention of the campaign has been to protect drinking water sources from contamination, which has been accomplished by deep well digging, by applying larvicides, and by filtering water through widely distributed nylon monofilament cloth filters. Educating communities about the guinea worm life cycle and transmission has been essential to the campaign. Mass media campaigns have engaged celebrities such as Miss Ghana to garner interest and collaboration in the local communities where guinea worm is prevalent. There is no better example of a community-based public health intervention than establishment of the guinea worm pond caretakers. These are typically respected, elderly men in their community who are no longer working their farms and have the time to sit and watch over the ponds where people collect water. Since water is typically collected by stepping into the pond or stream and filling plastic containers, caretakers examine the feet and ankles of anyone arriving to collect water. Pond caretakers ensure that nobody with guinea worm enters the water. If someone shows up and has the characteristic blister, the caretaker fetches the water for them.

Another key feature of the campaign is aggressive case containment and management. Anyone diagnosed with guinea worm (defined by strict case definition criteria) is taken to a case containment and management center until the person is fully treated. Assistance with any losses in work is provided as an incentive to stay at the center until treatment is complete. These centers are set up as camps with meals provided, and children and other family members are able to stay there as well. Removing the person with the active infection from the community also halts further transmission. Whenever a case of guinea worm is identified, active case surveillance can be conducted. Local public health workers do daily searches in the neighboring villages to identify additional cases. These measures do not require sophisticated technology, diagnostics, or medicine. Guinea worm eradication is one of the best examples of effective grassroots public health interventions, public health practice at its best.

By 2005, it was estimated that more than sixty-three million cases had been prevented and transmission stopped in more than half of the endemic countries. Today, there are just four remaining countries where guinea worm persists: South Sudan, Chad, Ethiopia, and Mali. [2] South Sudan is home to the majority of cases; eradication efforts there have been hindered by the long-term civil strife in that country. In the remaining three countries, incidence is down to fewer than a dozen cases reported each year.

Guinea-worm-free certification is given after an appropriate waiting period during which active surveillance in the country continues but does not reveal any new cases. Reducing the worldwide case burden to approximately 500 cases in just four countries from over 2.25 million cases in twenty-one countries when the program began in 1986 demonstrates the significant progress that has been made in a relatively short time.

The eradication campaign has not been without cost. The Bill and Melinda Gates Foundation and the British government have contributed the largest proportion of resources to this effort. The estimated cost per case is relatively low at $5 to $8, but the cumulative cost of the campaign—estimated at $225 million—has not been insignificant. It is well-known in public health that the last case or cases are always the most difficult and most costly to eliminate. Why? These last cases tend to be in the most challenging environments and where communities may be more difficult to organize due to war or civil unrest, greater distrust of public health authorities and/or international organizations, and extreme poverty.

Nonetheless, the progress in guinea worm eradication is notable. Guinea worm is poised to be the first disease to be eradicated without a medicine or vaccine. It will be eradicated as the result of

SIDEBAR 5-2

[____]

Nigeria's Last Case of Guinea Worm

Grace Otubo is famous in her Nigerian village. She is the last person in all of Nigeria to have contracted guinea worm. Nigeria, at one time the most endemic country for guinea worm disease in the world, has proudly declared victory in its twenty-year war against this parasite. Grace Otubo has shared how she kept herself from contracting guinea worm disease again, knowing that there is no vaccine or medicine to fight this disease. Instead she and her fellow community members had to change their living and drinking habits. She had to be convinced by health workers to drink only water filtered through a cloth that was provided to the villagers free of charge. Because the guinea worm larvae in the water are microscopic and it can be a year before infection is apparent, she and her fellow villagers had to adapt their behavior based on faith in what the public health officials were telling them. General Dr. Yakubu Gowon, former Nigerian head of state, was quoted as marking this important moment in Nigeria's history by saying, "we are staring history in the face as the public health system of Nigeria is about to make a bold statement of eradicating guinea worm disease in Nigeria after many years; over two decades of hard fought battle of guinea worm have now succeeded in defeating it."

From the Carter Center website (http://www.cartercenter.org/news/ features/h/guinea_worm/nigeria-last-gw.html).

solid and creative public health measures implemented by collaborating partners at every level.

GLOBAL EPIDEMIOLOGY OF HIV, TUBERCULOSIS, AND MALARIA

HIV, tuberculosis, and malaria: Even among lay people these three diseases are often recognized as important worldwide causes of morbidity and mortality from infectious diseases. These are the diseases that have been brought to light by high-profile celebrity crusades and far-reaching public awareness campaigns. It will be helpful to examine the epidemiology of these diseases to understand the impact in quantifiable terms and to understand the progress made in recent years, in large part due to the spotlight that has been turned on these three diseases.

Two measures of the impact from these diseases is the annual number of cases and deaths that they cause. The most recent data tell us there are an estimated 35 million people living with HIV worldwide, with approximately 2.5 million new infections occurring each year, or more than 6,000 new infections each day. An estimated 1.6 million people die as a result of HIV infection every year. [3] Infection with the bacteria that causes tuberculosis is much more common; if you lined up the world's population in single file, every third person would be infected with tuberculosis. Most would have the dormant form of infection rather than the active disease state. There are an estimated 8.6 million cases of tuberculosis each year, resulting in about 1.3 million deaths. [4] There is a large overlap in HIV and tuberculosis; many people suffer from both diseases.

To understand how widespread malaria is, consider that it is endemic in 104 of about 220 total countries in the world. This places about 40 percent of the world's population at risk for malaria. There are roughly 219 million malaria disease episodes each year and more than half a million deaths. [5] These deaths occur mostly in children under the age of five.

Global Epidemiology of HIV

The HIV pandemic has had a devastating impact on many families, communities, and nations. Fortunately, we have seen significant progress in reversing HIV global trends over the past decade. The vast majority, approximately twenty-five million of the thirty-five million people living with HIV, reside in sub-Saharan Africa. The South and Southeast Asia region is home to about four million people living with HIV, with much smaller numbers living in the remaining regions of the world. While the HIV pandemic is concentrated in southern Africa, it is not evenly distributed across Africa. Not surprisingly, most of the deaths from HIV occur where the burden is the greatest.

The HIV epidemic has shortened life expectancy in the African countries that have been hardest hit by the disease. Life expectancy for countries such as Botswana, South Africa, Swaziland, Zambia, and Zimbabwe had started to reach the sixth decade in the late 1980s and early 1990s, but it plummeted once HIV spread. Fortunately, we have seen a reversal of this trend in many countries, with life expectancy beginning to rise, hopefully to return to the pre-HIV epidemic levels.

Of the more than six thousand new HIV infections each day, about 95 percent of these are occurring in low- to middle-income countries. While most of these are in adults, about seven hundred are in children under the age of fifteen, almost exclusively through mother-to-child transmission.

HIV, not surprisingly, is still a global health priority. Rather than associate the HIV burden with an entire continent, however, it is important to appreciate the geographic variation across continents and countries. The absolute number of infected individuals continues to rise; in fact the number of new infections exceeds the number of deaths each year. While a decrease in the number of new infections is an important goal of HIV control, the lowered mortality is the benefit of increased access to HIV treatment. The HIV pandemic is well established now in every country with some variations in intensity, modes of transmission, access to treatment, and the access and success of preventive approaches. It has been a challenge to address the underlying health care inequities that have hindered access to care and implementation of the most effective preventive measures.

In 2007, UNAIDS issued a press release claiming that the global HIV prevalence had leveled off. Specifically, HIV prevalence in 2007 had decreased to an estimated 33 million people living with HIV from an estimated 38 million in 2006. Similarly, the estimated number of new infections was reduced from 4.1 million in 2006 to 2.5 million in 2007. And lastly, deaths were also estimated to have decreased from 2.8 million in 2006 to 2.1 million in 2007. [6]

How did UNAIDS account for these dramatic changes in the HIV data? The efforts to scale up HIV prevention activities could not explain the sharp decline in these figures in just one year's time. Rather, this downward revision in HIV data was largely due to expanded surveillance data collection and improved methodologies. Data such as the numbers of cases, deaths, and new infections are determined through surveys and reviews of existing data and extrapolation from these representative samples. In this particular case, about 70 percent of the decrease in prevalence data came from changes in the data from India and five sub-Saharan African countries. The more accurate surveillance data provided more reliable estimates, therefore the previous years' higher estimates were, to some extent, due to surveillance artifact. In some countries, of course, there were actual declines in prevalence, most notably Zimbabwe, Cote d'Ivoire, and Kenya. Such declines in prevalence are clearly an improvement in the overall control of the

HIV pandemic, though in some areas, or "pockets," prevalence rates remain quite high.

It is important to understand the relationship between prevalence, incidence, and mortality. In areas where the prevalence rate is stable, what does that tell us about the epidemic? A stable prevalence rate may give the appearance that an epidemic is under control when it may not be. Prevalence is the mathematical product of incidence multiplied by the duration of disease. Therefore, a stable prevalence can result when the disease incidence increases but the duration of the disease decreases; in other words, there may be increased transmission and a concomitant increase in mortality (since a high death rate shortens the duration of the disease). Prevalence can increase when incidence stays constant but the duration of the disease is lengthened due to greater access to noncurative treatment (such as the medications available for HIV infection). A curative therapy would shorten the duration of the disease, which would decrease prevalence if incidence were unchanged. Therefore, a stable, or even increasing, prevalence rate can mask the changes in incidence and mortality, making it impossible to determine whether this is a desirable effect or trend without further information.

The improved data collection between 2006 and 2007 also resulted in a decrease in estimated HIV incidence, with the greatest decline occurring in sub-Saharan Africa and South and Southeast Asia. Incidence is a figure that is estimated, not directly measured. Given the mathematical relationship between incidence, prevalence, and duration of disease, a decrease in prevalence (measured and extrapolated) coupled with an increase in duration of disease (due to improved access to life-prolonging antiretrovirals) results in a decrease in incidence. Understanding this relationship is important to be able to accurately interpret epidemiologic data.

Global Epidemiology of Malaria

There are four species of the plasmodium that causes malaria: falciparum, vivax, ovale, and knowlesi. The vast majority of deaths are caused by falciparum malaria. The number of estimated malaria cases worldwide peaked at 244 million in 2005; in 2010, the year for which we have the most recent data, it had decreased to 219 million cases. [5] All WHO regions are reporting decreases in the number of malaria cases, and the global incidence of malaria fell 17 percent between 2000 and 2010. Deaths are also decreasing; there were nearly a million malaria deaths in 2000, but by 2010 that number had been cut nearly in half, to 550,000 deaths. In that year, for the first time, the European region reported no cases of malaria, and nine countries were taking the next step of implementing elimination programs. Another eight countries were in the pre-elimination stage, gearing up for entering full-blown elimination programming. Many countries are reporting decreases in cases, in the number of hospital admissions for malaria, and in deaths since 2000.

This disease primarily strikes two already vulnerable populations, namely children and pregnant women. Malaria is a leading cause of mortality in children under the age of five and is responsible for almost one-fifth of all deaths in this age group. In sub-Saharan Africa, pregnant women are also disproportionately affected and can have adverse outcomes and sequelae such as perinatal mortality, low birth weight in the infant, and severe anemia in the mother.

Drug resistance is an important challenge that has been thwarting malaria treatment and control efforts for decades. Resistance to one of the oldest drugs for malaria, chloroquine, is now widespread and resulted in a doubling of malaria deaths among children under the age of five between 1990 and 1998. There is currently no vaccine available for malaria, though there are several candidates being evaluated. The results of a phase 3 clinical trial of the RTS,S/ASO1 candidate vaccine showed modest protection in preventing clinical malaria in infants. [7] Pending further evaluation of its safety and efficacy, this vaccine may be available in a few years, likely targeted for use in high-risk populations. There are four key interventions currently in use to control malaria: (1) insecticide-treated bed nets; (2) artemisinin-based combination therapies (ACTS), the highly effective combination therapies that are now being used to treat the otherwise resistant strains of malaria; (3) indoor residual spraying of insecticides inside people's houses; and (4) intermittent presumptive therapy for malaria, which is the treatment of certain high-risk groups, such as pregnant women, at specific intervals without requiring any testing. Presumptive treatment is done in settings with few resources where the risk of disease outweighs the risk of the treatment. Implementation of this intervention is relatively simple if the drugs are available. Treatment and prevention of malaria are discussed in greater detail in chapter 9.

Global Epidemiology of Tuberculosis

It was in 1993, now more than twenty years ago, when the World Health Organization took the unprecedented step of declaring TB a global emergency. Because of concerted efforts on a global, national, and community level, the number of new TB cases has been declining for the past several years. The countries with the largest populations, India and China, bear the greatest burden of TB cases in terms of absolute numbers, and are home to approximately 40 percent of the world's TB patients. Another 24 percent of the world's TB patients live in an African country. The African and European regions have not experienced the same degree of success as the rest of the world, maintaining similar or sometimes even higher rates of TB compared to their 1990 levels. While many factors may explain this slow progress, there is no doubt that drug resistance in the European region and the HIV epidemic in the African region have played important roles.

As with the distribution of HIV infection, sub-Saharan Africa as a region shoulders the greatest burden, but Africa is not a homogeneous continent. For example, Tanzania in East Africa is one country whose successful TB program has lowered its TB rate from 236 per 100,000 to 165 per 100,000 between the years of 2000 and 2012. [4] Several other African countries such as Botswana and Ghana have cut their TB rates in half over the same time period. [4] While we often think about TB and HIV by region, it is more accurate to consider these disease burdens on a country-by-country basis.

Drug resistance has been a major factor impeding TB control, even outside the European region. There were an estimated 450,000 new cases of multidrug-resistant TB, or MDR TB, worldwide in 2012. [4] The vast majority of cases were confined to just twenty-seven high-burden countries. [4] Unfortunately, only a small proportion of all TB cases are tested for drug resistance. Less than 25 percent of the estimated patients with drug-resistant TB were detected in 2012. [4] In 2006, we saw the emergence of what is now termed extensively-drug-resistant TB, or XDR TB. This strain of TB is resistant to several classes of first-line and second-line medicines, making it difficult to treat. At least one case of XDR TB has been reported from nearly half the countries in the world. [4]

The HIV pandemic has been an important driver of the TB epidemic, especially in sub-Saharan Africa. About 75 percent of the estimated 1.1 million patients with TB/HIV codisease reside in the African region. [4] When TB data from high HIV prevalent African countries are examined separately from those with a low HIV prevalence rate, there is a clear relationship between rates of TB and HIV. On average, about 40 percent of TB patients in the African region are HIV-infected. In some countries like Swaziland, this rate is as high as 77 percent. [4] Recent pushes for expanded HIV testing among TB patients and screening of HIV patients for TB has resulted in nearly half of all TB patients knowing their HIV status; this indicator jumps to 74 percent when considering TB patients in the African region.

CONCLUSION

Understanding key epidemiology and surveillance terms and concepts is essential to appreciating the impact that infectious diseases are having on our population worldwide. Further, this understanding is critical to designing effective control efforts so we can move toward elimination and eventually eradication. While it can be difficult to digest so many facts and figures when discussing infectious disease epidemiology, one must remember that behind every statistic is a human being whose life has been cut short or irrevocably altered by disease. For those working on the frontlines of care, it is the human face that remains the most prominent. Our team in Tanzania often draws upon the words of a colleague who worked during the early days of the HIV epidemic in Dar es Salaam. She always remarked that if statistics are numbers with the tears washed off them, we are dealing with the tears.

REFERENCES

1. McNeill WH. Plagues and peoples. Anchor Books: New York, 1998.

2. The Carter Center website, Guinea worm case countdown. http://www.cartercenter.org/health/guinea_worm/mini_site/current.html, accessed December 3, 2013.

3. Joint United Nations Programme on HIV/AIDS (UNAIDS). Global report: UNAIDS report on the global AIDS epidemic 2013. Geneva, UNAIDS, 2013.

4. World Health Organization. Global tuberculosis report 2013;

WHO report 2013. Geneva: World Health Organization, WHO/HTM/ TB/2013.11.

5. World Health Organization. World malaria report: 2012. Geneva: World Health Organization.

6. Joint United Nations Programme on HIV/AIDS and World Health Organization. AIDS epidemic update: December 2007. Geneva: Joint United Nations Programme on HIV/AIDS and World Health Organization, UNAIDS/07.27E/JC1322E.

7. The RTS,S Clinical Trials Partnership. A Phase 3 Trial of RTS,S/ AS01 Malaria Vaccine in African Infants. 2012 Dec 13;367(24):2284–95.

6

THE BASIC NECESSITIES OF LIFE

Nutrition, Water, and Sanitation

John R. Butterly

A hungry man is not a free man

— Adlai Stevenson

Chronic hunger and malnutrition are at the forefront of the problems facing the people of the developing nations: hence Goal #1 of the Millennium Development Goals: eradicate extreme poverty and hunger. While it remains controversial whether or not there is such a thing as a poverty trap, as stated by Jeffrey Sachs [1], the director of the Earth Institute at Columbia University and the special advisor to the United Nations Secretary-General on the Millennium Development Goals, we think it is fair to say that should such a trap exist, chronic hunger and malnutrition are the locks on that trap. Chronic and persistent food insecurity and the resultant malnutrition robs an individual of the ability to develop his or her full potential and robs a society of its most important resource: its human capital. A full discussion of the physical and mental effects chronic malnutrition has in stunting the physical, intellectual, and emotional growth of a person is beyond the scope of this chapter. In this chapter we review the basic science of nutrition, define the different forms of malnutrition associated with macronutrient deficiency, and discuss the effects this has in compromising our ability to fight off disease.

We divide nutrients into two general categories, micronutrients and macronutrients. Micronutrients include the vitamins, both water-soluble such as the B vitamin complex and vitamin C as well as the fat-soluble vitamins A, D, E, and K. Also included in the micronutrients are a number of inorganic minerals such as iron and iodine. These substances are essential for our health and well-being even though they are needed only in trace amounts in our diet. Inadequate dietary intake of these micronutrients leads to specific health issues, but the only one we will address here is vitamin A deficiency because of its substantial effect on mortality rates in children under the age of five years.

The macronutrients are divided into three basic categories: carbohydrates, lipids or fats, and protein. The carbohydrates include sugars such as sucrose (table sugar) and lactose (milk sugar) and starch (called amylase if a plant source, glycogen if animal). The basic formula of carbohydrates is a carbon connected to two hydrogen atoms and an oxygen atom. Of course, two hydrogen atoms and an oxygen atom are a molecule of water, hence hydrated carbon or carbohydrate. Carbohydrates supply four calories per gram. Dietary calories are actually kilocalories; one calorie is the energy it takes to raise the temperature of one cubic centimeter of water one degree centigrade. For the purposes of this discussion, we will use the commonly understood meaning of the word "calories." Carbohydrates are the basic source of energy or ATP (Adenosine triphosphate), a high-energy molecule that our cells use for life's functions. They can be stored to some extent as the animal starch glycogen, but require substantial water to be stored with them, so this is not a very efficient means for us to store excess energy. The fats or lipids include triglycerides and cholesterol. Fats have the highest energy content. While carbohydrates have four calories per gram, energy-dense fats have nine calories per gram. In addition to this, fats are hydrophobic so they can be stored without water. For these reasons, excess nutrients are stored as fats in adipose tissue, so fats can be used both as a rich energy source as well as an efficient means of excess energy storage. Protein also has four calories per gram but is generally not used as an energy source. In the normally fed state, we preferentially recycle about 75 percent of the amino acids derived from our ingested protein to build other proteins. The reason for this is that there are ten amino acids out of the naturally occurring twenty that we cannot synthesize in our bodies. These are called essential amino acids. As we take in these essential amino acids as protein in our diet, it is critical that we are able to recycle them so that we can build proteins necessary for our own bodies to function. This is a fundamental point in understanding the biological repercussions of inadequate nutrition and the particularly insidious damage done by inadequate protein in the diet.

We tend to think of DNA, the nucleic acid found in the nuclei of cells, as the central biomolecule of life. It is self-replicating, self-repairing, and codes for all the information that makes you "you," but DNA is only potential life, and it is not until DNA is translated into protein that one can actually function as a living organism. Proteins are how we move, how we communicate internally, and how we translate genetic information into form and function.

For this reason, when we talk about malnutrition, we define it as protein-energy malnutrition, the definition of which is that the body's need for protein, energy fuel, or both are not satisfied by diet. There can be a wide spectrum of clinical manifestations depending on whether there is a pure protein deficit versus an energy deficit or both, and clinical variables include the severity of malnutrition, duration, what has caused it, the age of the individual, and whether or not there are other deficits such as vitamin deficiencies or infection.

We can classify protein-energy malnutrition as primary when it is due to inadequate food intake, or as secondary protein-energy malnutrition, which can be the result of a disease that leads to decreased food intake, decreased absorption, or increased requirements. Examples of the latter may be seen in patients with AIDS, certain cancers, and tuberculosis.

If the primary nutrient deficiency is energy, the clinical syndrome is called *marasmus,* a word that comes from the Greek word for withering. If on the other hand, the primary deficiency is inadequate protein intake, we see a disease in which the individual becomes swollen due to fluid retention or edema, and this is called *kwashiorkor.* This word comes from the Ga tribe in Ghana and loosely translates as the disease the first child gets when the second child is born. This is a perfect way to describe this disease; when the second child is born, the first child is weaned from breast milk, and when breast milk is the only source of high-quality protein available to a child of only one to two years of age and is replaced by a diet high in carbohydrates (essentially "empty calories," lacking in essential amino acids), severe protein malnutrition results.

Protein-energy malnutrition is the most important nutritional disease in developing nations. It has a high prevalence, it is related to high child mortality, and it leads to serious child morbidity causing impaired physical growth as well as inadequate social and intellectual development. Most malnourished, and by this we mean *undernourished* people, live in developing countries.

According to the most recent report from the UN's Food and Agricultural Organization (FAO) in 2013, 842 million people, or one in eight of the world's population, are chronically hungry and undernourished. [2] The vast majority of these people live in developing countries. While the largest number of these individuals live in Asia, remember the potential for misleading statistics; the populations in Asian countries are much larger than in sub-Saharan Africa. If we were to look at the *percent* of populations that are malnourished in these countries, sub-Saharan Africa would top the list. Of course, primary protein-energy malnutrition is seen in the United States as well, generally in vulnerable populations, such as children in lower socioeconomic groups, the elderly who live alone, and adults with substance abuse problems such as alcohol abuse and drug addiction. These are not the only individuals suffering from chronic malnutrition and food insecurity in the United States, however. At the time of this writing, an average of 14 percent of the populations in each of the fifty states is food insecure. [3]

THE SPECIAL CASE OF PROTEIN AND KWASHIORKOR

We should take some time to discuss the mechanism of the development of kwashiorkor because it underlines the importance of protein in the diet. As an individual undergoes a progressive negative energy balance, there are adaptive mechanisms. From the perspective of energy deficiency, an individual can compensate substantially by decreasing the level of energy expended in what might be considered discretionary activities: work in adults and play in children. There are a number of metabolic adaptations that occur as well, but the one we are most interested in here is that of protein metabolism.

Normally we recycle 75 percent of ingested amino acids. The recycled amino acids are used for protein synthesis, while 25 percent is broken down for metabolic purposes, usually to make "new" glucose through the process called gluconeogenesis. If there is enough high-quality protein in the diet (protein with significant amounts of essential amino acids), the individual can adapt and increase the recycled amount of amino acids to 90 to 95 percent so that critical proteins in the body can be synthesized and nondiscretionary activity, that is, visceral function, can be preserved.

Individuals suffering from this level of protein energy malnutrition undergo skeletal muscle wasting with sparing of the visceral or organ proteins. This is the clinical syndrome of marasmus. A person with marasmus will appear extremely thin and wasted, but the person's internal organs will be working normally. Because of this, in a basal or resting state, basal oxygen consumption per kilogram of body weight will actually increase because more body weight is made up of functioning vital organs as opposed to resting skeletal muscle. This cannot happen in kwashiorkor. Because of the absence of essential amino acids, adaptation to increased recycling of protein cannot occur; the body cannibalizes not only skeletal muscle but also the muscles of the vital organs. Because of this, basal oxygen consumption per kilogram body weight will actually decrease because the organs are not functioning normally. It is easy to see why this is a particularly dangerous form of malnutrition. Organ failure occurs earlier, mortality rates are high, and recovery of those suffering from kwashiorkor, usually children, is more difficult.

One can easily appreciate the difference in appearance between kwashiorkor and marasmus. People who have marasmus have the typical appearance one would associate with extreme undernutrition; a wasted look with total loss of body fat and near total loss of skeletal muscle—a true "skin and bones" appearance. A person (usually a child) on the other hand, by superficial examination appears chubby. This is misleading as the puffiness of the face and the protuberance of the belly and swelling of the legs is actually fluid accumulation and dilation of loops of bowel in the abdomen because the smooth muscle in the wall of the intestines is no longer working. The one look victims of marasmus and kwashiorkor have in common is an unmistakable look of pain and fear—understandable under the circumstances. People affected by malnutrition are usually the most vulnerable, which means children and women.

In order to make the diagnosis of malnutrition, it is important to use simple, accurate, and sensitive measurements that are available in the field and that have an existing reference standard. It would not do to bring a large and expensive machine into an un-

TABLE 6-1

INDEX	Clinical Status	Normal (% of median)	Mild (% of median)	Moderate (% of median)	Severe (% of median)
Weight for height	Wasting	90–110	80–89	70–79	<70
Height for age	Stunting	95–105	90–94	85–89	<85

derdeveloped field situation where a malfunction would cause an inability to bring help to these people. It is for this reason that we use basic anthropometric measurements such as height and weight.

Two indices used for basic measures in children include weight for height, which is an index for current nutritional status, and height for age, which is an index for past nutritional history. These indices define the clinical status of a child, with *wasting* being a term that describes a deficit in weight for height and *stunting* defining height-for-age.

Table 6-1 shows examples and levels of malnutrition, either due to wasting or stunting. The number is given as a median so that these can be normalized depending on regional variability.

The metric used in adults is that of body mass index, which is defined as weight in kilograms divided by height in meters squared. While we are talking about undernutrition, we define malnutrition as more or less severe depending on a body mass index of less than 18.5, while the malnutrition associated with nutritional diseases of affluence are more along the other end of the spectrum, defining overweight as BMI>25, obesity as BMI>30, and morbid obesity as BMI>40.

In summary, protein-energy malnutrition is a continuum of deficit based on the degree, duration, characteristics of the patient, and specific nutritional deficit. Two distinct entities of nutritional

TABLE 6-2

BMI	PEM
18.5	Normal
17–18.4	Mild
16–16.9	Moderate
<16	Severe

deficiency include marasmus, which is primarily an energy deficit, and kwashiorkor, which is primarily a protein deficit. One can see a mixed picture as well. The detail of the pathophysiology is an important medical problem, but of course the fact that this occurs at all is an imperative social problem. This is why ending hunger and extreme poverty is the first goal of the millennium development project.

VITAMIN A

There are nine water-soluble vitamins (the Bcomplex vitamins and vitamin C) and four fat-soluble vitamins (A, D, E, and K). All of these are vitally important in our diets (the term vitamin is a conjugation of the words "vital" and "amine" as the first of these to be discovered were all members of a chemical family known as amines). The absence of any one of these essential nutrients in our diet is accompanied by the development of specific, potentially fatal disease states. We will only discuss vitamin A deficiency in depth here since it is so commonly associated with chronic protein energy malnutrition and a fundamental underlying cause of morbidity and mortality in malnourished populations, especially in children under the age of five.

Vitamin A is found in both animal and vegetable tissues. The form of vitamin A found in meat is generally in the form of retinol or retinoic acid. These forms are extremely bioavailable and active forms of vitamin A. In addition, because vitamin A is fat-soluble, it requires adequate fat in the diet for significant amounts to be absorbed. Diets rich in animal protein are generally also rich in fat, so animal sources of vitamin A are highly desirable, both because the vitamin A is in active form and because it is easily absorbed due to the relatively high fat content of the associated meal. Vegetable sources of vitamin A are generally the yellow or orange vegetables such as carrots, sweet potatoes, and squash, as well as some leafy green vegetables. The vitamin A in these sources is actually a provitamin, a group of organic molecules known as carotenoids, the most important one being beta-carotene. These provitamins must be converted intracellularly to the active vitamin A and do not supply the same amount of vitamin A as do retinol and retinoic acid. In addition, diets high in vegetable sources of vitamin A are generally much lower in fat, so that actual absorption of the compounds is adversely affected.

Vitamin A is necessary for normal vision (as the name of the active form—retinol—might suggest). Retinol is necessary for the production of rhodopsin, the active photosensitive pigment in the retina necessary for vision. Inadequate vitamin A in the diet will lead to night blindness and eventual total blindness through the following mechanism. Vitamin A is also critically important for the development of healthy epithelial tissue. In addition to breakdown of the mucous membranes, which may allow entry of pathogenic organisms through these primary barriers of defense in cases of vitamin A deficiency, more worrisome is that this deficiency leads to ulceration, infection, and scarring of the cornea in affected individuals. In situations where the vitamin A deficiency is chronic, this leads to eventual total blindness due to the corneal scarring and retinal dysfunction. In fact, vitamin A deficiency is the number one cause of preventable blindness in children worldwide. [4]

In addition to its function in normal vision and cell development, vitamin A is critical for the normal functioning of the immune system. It is for this reason that vitamin-A-deficient individuals, especially children, are more susceptible to infection by any pathogens, both those that are primary pathogens as well as those that would be considered opportunistic. This is also why these infections are more severe and more likely to lead to prolonged disability or death. For example, it is estimated that two-thirds of the preventable deaths in children under the age of five are due directly or indirectly to vitamin A deficiency. [5] While it is estimated that there are 250 million preschool children worldwide who are deficient in vitamin A, and that between 250,000 and 500,000 children a year become blind due to this deficiency, we should be aware that adequate vitamin A intake can be made available to large populations for pennies a day and that such vitamin supplementation has made great inroads in decreasing mortality rates in children (and pregnant women) by 23 percent overall and 50 percent in cases of acute measles. [4]

STARVATION AND SUSCEPTIBILITY TO DISEASE

If you recall, chapter 3 began with a quote from Sir William Osler, "humanity has but three great enemies: fever, famine and war. Of these by far the greatest, by far the most terrible, is fever." During the remainder of this chapter, you will come understand why this is so. We will talk briefly about some of the historical diseases associated with chronic malnutrition, and later in this book we will discuss more contemporary diseases that plague us.

Recall that we define virulence as the degree of the capacity of an organism to cause disease. Host characteristics (such as malnutrition) as well as intrinsic virulence are important in determining whether or not disease occurs and how severe that disease is. In this section we will also address microbial encounter and entry and avoidance of host defenses.

Microbial encounter and entry become increasingly likely as people suffer conditions associated with poverty or conflict. The overcrowding one sees in such situations, in addition to increasing the likelihood of transmission of infections from person to person, is also associated with either primary lack of infrastructure or breakdown of existing infrastructure, which can then lead to poor hygiene, inadequate sanitation, and contamination of existing water supplies. In these settings, infectious agents are increasingly encountered and easily gain entry into people's bodies either through contamination of the water supply, contamination of food or the physical environment (fomites), or in some cases through transmission by insect vectors (e.g., mosquitoes, lice, and fleas).

We have multiple, complex immunological systems we use to fight off infections. While these functions are extremely effective in intact and healthy people, individuals who are chronically malnourished have compromised immune systems. As we noted earlier, microbes are generally more frequently encountered by these individuals because of the lack of infrastructure (safe sanitation and safe water supplies) associated with populations that are malnourished. In addition, the physical barriers (skin, mucous membranes) begin to break down and internal protective mechanisms begin to fail. The overall consequence is that of a greater predisposition to infection with more severe complications in a situation that would otherwise be a minor infection (or no infection at all) in a well-fed population. This is what is meant by the term "opportunistic infections in compromised hosts."

THE TRADITIONAL DISEASES ASSOCIATED WITH WIDESPREAD CHRONIC MALNUTRITION

The epidemic diseases associated with populations subjected to chronic malnutrition are those linked to inadequate resources in the form of public health infrastructure; they include scarlet fever, diphtheria, dysentery, cholera, typhus, typhoid fever, and tuberculosis. For the purposes of this section, we will briefly discuss dysentery, cholera, typhus, and typhoid fever. Tuberculosis is discussed in detail in chapter 8.

Dysentery

Dysentery, which means disease of the bowel, is a disorder of the large intestines characterized by inflammation, abdominal pain, and frequent stools containing blood, pus, and mucus. There may or may not be significant diarrhea. The term itself was first used by Hippocrates to describe this very clinical scenario, but of course the etiology was not clearly defined until the end of the nineteenth century with the development of the germ theory of disease and identification of the two major causes of dysentery (bacillary, which we will discuss briefly here, and amebic, which we will not discuss). The prototypic organism for invasive bacterial dysentery is an organism called Shigella, a bacteria related to E. coli. Accurate data is not readily available to determine the true epidemiology of this disease, but it is estimated that 165 million cases occur annually worldwide, with 100 million of these occurring in developing nations. Annual mortality is estimated at one million, and the highest rate of infection (up to 70 percent of cases) and highest mortality (60 percent of all deaths) occur in children less than five years of age. [6] While breastfeeding infants, even in developing nations, are resistant to Shigella dysentery, probably due to isolation from contaminated water and food supplies, it is also true that disease rates, severity of illness, and complications are closely associated with the severity of accompanying malnutrition. Mortality is unusual except in malnourished children and older adults. [7]

The mode of infection with this organism is transmission from fecal-oral spread or contaminated water supply. Ingested bacteria pass through the stomach and small intestine and invade the lining of the large intestine by means of an invasion virulence factor. The organism spreads locally from cell to cell, and because of a virulence factor known as a Shiga toxin, it is able to damage and destroy the cells lining the large bowel. In the well-fed adult, this disease may remain self-limited to a nonbloody, watery diarrhea. Compromised individuals are much more likely to develop the full-blown systemic disease, and children are especially likely to develop serious, invasive disease.

Extra intestinal complications, the majority of which arise in developing countries, can occur, in part due to the prevalence of more virulent strains but also related to the poor nutritional status of the host. An example of this is bacteremia, an invasion of the bloodstream with the bacteria. Bacteremia is associated with a higher mortality and is more common in children less than one year of age and in people with protein-energy malnutrition. The treatment for this disease is complex and depends on the strain of bacteria, ability to rehydrate the patient, presence of a safe water supply, appropriate antibiotic therapy (although multiple drug resistance is seen), and possibly surgery if there is enough destruction of the tissues or abscess formation. A much more effective—albeit more complex—way to deal with this is through prevention, with improved sanitation, safe water supplies, and improved nutrition.

Cholera

Another enteric disease associated with poor nutrition and inadequate infrastructure is cholera. The term cholera comes from a Greek word meaning a flow of bile. It was first described as a distinct entity in 1817. There have been seven pandemics in the modern era, the first six between 1817 and 1923. Cholera is caused by a curved bacillus, *Vibrio cholera*, which was first described in the stool of victims in 1854 and again in 1883 by Robert Koch. The organism is particularly dangerous in that it can live in aquatic environments attached to algae and small shrimp-like organisms called copepods. It can survive for years in that environment with no human hosts and remain dormant so that it cannot be cultured. As you will recall, in chapter 4, we discussed the first epidemiologic study by John Snow in London, which demonstrated that cholera was transmitted by water.

Cholera has some unique features in its epidemiology. It has a predisposition to cause epidemics with pandemic potential, in part due to its virulence, as well as its ability to contaminate water supplies. In addition, because of its ability to remain dormant, it is able to remain endemic in all affected areas. Cholera can be transmitted from an index case infected from water or food and is known to have been transmitted through rice, raw fish, seafood, raw oysters, and fresh fruits. There have even been cases of transmission during funerals in Africa reportedly from people touching a nondisinfected corpse and then eating. [8]

Vibrio cholera is the prototype for noninvasive bacterial diarrhea. Cholera toxin, as we discussed in chapter 3, is an exotoxin and is secreted exteriorly to the bacteria. It acts to increase levels of cyclic AMP in the cells lining the small intestine, which inhibits absorption of sodium and causes secretion of chloride. Water from the body then follows passively, causing copious watery diarrhea, which is so watery it is described as rice water stools. This causes varying degrees of dehydration, which occurs rapidly and can be severe. Mortality rates can be as high as 10 percent with fetal loss in pregnant women as high as 50 percent. With proper treatment, mortality can be lower than 1 percent. Rehydration is the key to treatment. Antibiotic therapy is actually secondary although it may decrease the time needed for rehydration and hospitalization. As is true of dysentery, the key is prevention through adequate sanitation facilities, protection of the water supply, and good hygiene.

Typhus

Typhus is a classic disease of famine and war, and unlike most of the diseases we have discussed, it is transmitted via an insect vector. Many of the pioneering scientists who worked on typhus, including Howard Taylor Ricketts and Stanislaus von Prowazek, contracted typhus themselves and died. Charles Nicole, the only survivor of the early work, was awarded the Nobel Prize in 1923 for demonstrating that the vector was the body louse. Occurrence of typhus in the past one hundred years parallels the history of war and famine, with thirty million cases recorded in the Soviet Union in the years 1918 through 1922, and an estimated three million deaths.

An interesting historical anecdote occurred during World War II, when there was an extremely high attack rate in the concentration camps due to the deplorable overcrowding and lack of hygiene. Because it would be extremely debilitating to German troops (Napoleon lost close to 400,000 of the soldiers of his Grande Armee of 500,000 to typhus during his attack on Moscow in 1812), the German army went out of its way to avoid areas of epidemic typhus. To avoid these areas, the German army was preceded by a group of doctors who tested the population using a special test called the Weil-Felix reaction, which cross-reacts with typhus. A group of Polish physicians knew this and vaccinated individuals with a cross-reacting organism to create an artificial epidemic area and keep the German army out.

There are two forms of the disease: primary typhus, which was distinguished from typhoid fever in 1836, and a recurrent or recrudescent form known as Brill's disease, which is milder and not associated with body lice. Recrudescent disease occurs when an individual who has had typhus has a relapse due to activation of dormant organisms in his system, and the organism once again appears in the person's blood. The primary disease is transmitted through the bite of the body louse, which transmits the organism *Rickettsia prowazekii,* named for Ricketts and Prowazek, two of the original investigators. The louse feeds on a person with Rickettsia in his or her blood. A large number of these organisms appear in the louse feces within one week. When the louse feeds on another individual, it defecates, and if the individual scratches the bite (which is inevitable), the rickettsia-laden feces is rubbed into the wound. The organism will then grow locally and spread throughout the bloodstream, invading cells lining the small blood vessels (it is an obligate intracellular pathogen; remember that term from chapter 3 on infectious disease). This can cause dysfunction and death of the affected tissue.

Typhus is common in winter and during civil conflict, when clothing is not changed frequently, there is crowding of individuals, and infrastructure for hygiene is unavailable. While untreated typhus will resolve after two weeks, it is followed by a long convalescence of two to three months, and mortality rates can be as high as 40 percent, especially among the senior population. The treatment is relatively simple, as the disease is sensitive to antibiotics and responds to a single dose of the tetracycline/doxycycline, but the best way to control typhus is by prevention via sanitation, good hygiene, and delousing of the population.

Typhoid fever

Typhoid fever was initially confused with typhus; hence, the similar name. It is caused by a totally different bacteria called salmonella, a genus named after Daniel E. Salmon, who was awarded one of the first degrees as doctor of veterinary medicine from the Cornell School of Veterinary Medicine and who served as the chief of the Bureau of Animal Industry in the U.S. Department of Agriculture. This organism is unrelated to the rickettsial organism that causes typhus, but is a member of the same family as E. coli and is found widely in nature and in the gastrointestinal tracts of domestic and wild mammals, reptiles, birds, and insects.

Salmonella typhi and Salmonella paratyphi (the species of salmonella that cause typhoid fever) are pathogens only in humans. They are highly effective human pathogens, but limited in the species they can affect. The disease can be acquired only through close contact with a person who has had typhoid fever or is a chronic carrier. As is true of so many of the diseases associated with inadequate infrastructure and usually occurring in regions where chronic malnutrition is widespread, typhoid fever is an enteric infection spread by exposure to contaminated food or water.

Typhoid fever has continued to be a global health problem; the WHO estimated sixteen million cases and 600,000 deaths annually worldwide in 1994, and the most recent estimates from the Center for Disease Control and the WHO estimate between twenty million and twenty-five million cases annually in 2004 to present. [9] It is epidemic in many developing regions such as India, South and Central America, Africa, and Asia. These areas have the shared characteristics of rapid population growth, increased urbanization, inadequate human waste treatment, and overburdened health care systems.

Pathogenesis starts with ingestion of the organisms causing invasion of the bowel wall and a primary bacteremia. Bacteria are ingested by the mononuclear phagocytes that we discussed earlier in the chapter. Ironically, typhoid is a disease of the very cells meant to destroy them, as the bacteria multiply intracellularly, where they are protected from other aspects of the immune system. When the intracellular organisms reach a critical threshold, they destroy the cell they are in, and secondary bacteremia occurs. This time they establish themselves in the gallbladder of the infected individual and invade the lymphoid tissue in the intestine and lymph nodes. Because they are in the gallbladder, the organisms are excreted back into the intestine and can then be excreted into the environment.

In chapter 3, we mentioned the possibility of gene mutations occurring and persisting in populations that may be exposed to frequent infections in endemic areas. Cystic fibrosis is caused by an abnormality in what is called the cystic fibrosis transmembrane conduction regulator or CFTR. Homozygous individuals are born with life-shortening disease and do not reproduce. There is, however, a persistent gene frequency of 4 to 5 percent heterozygotes in European populations that have historically been exposed to high rates of infection with *Salmonella typhi* and *paratyphi*. It happens that *Salmonella typhi* uses this same membrane protein (CFTR) as a receptor to enter the gastrointestinal submucosa, that is, the virulence factor that codes for the invasive behavior in *Salmonella typhi* that enables it to adhere to this membrane receptor. It is believed that heterozygotes might have a selective advantage due to decreased susceptibility to *Salmonella typhi* because the organism is not able to attach to the abnormal membrane receptor and therefore is unable to gain entry into the host. Because typhoid fever can colonize the gallbladder and otherwise remain silent, one can see chronic asymptomatic carriers. These have generally been over the age of fifty and have usually been women with gallstones. In these patients, *Salmonella typhi* can live in the bile and gallstones and be excreted into the small intestine with the bile. The most famous of these cases occurred in the early 1900s, with a woman named Mary Mallon, known as Typhoid Mary. She emigrated from Ireland and was a cook for a number of families. She never realized that she had typhoid fever and in fact never believed it. It was only after a number of people for whom she cooked died that it was recognized that she was an asymptomatic carrier of the disease (a state that had been previously unreported in the medical literature). She was told to stop working as a cook, but because she refused to believe that she carried the disease she changed her name and continued to seek out jobs as a cook, infecting more people. Eventually she was involuntarily quarantined, the first incidence of involuntary quarantine of an otherwise healthy individual in the United States.

The disease itself is manifested as an acute systemic febrile illness with an incubation time depending on how many organisms were ingested. The hallmark of typhoid fever is a persistent fever of four to eight weeks in an untreated patient. Abdominal symptoms may be mild and near asymptomatic or fulminant and not necessarily associated with diarrhea. Three to five percent of patients become asymptomatic chronic carriers, some for life. Unfortunately, treatment with the use of antibiotics may lead to a high relapse rate: 20 percent compared to 5 to 10 percent in untreated patients. Once again, prevention with improvement in sanitation and protection of the water supply is the best means of protecting the population.

WATER AND SANITATION

Thousands have lived without love,
Not one without water.
—*W. H. Auden*

In order to understand the fundamental importance of access to potable water and sanitation to the basic health and well-being of individuals and populations, it is important to know the characteristics of water, both physical and chemical, as they apply to all living organisms. We should also understand the important geographical issues, as well as the demographics of access to safe water supplies, adequate sanitation, and the effects they have on health and hygiene.

Earth has been called the water planet. There are 332,500,000 cubic miles of water on the earth. Putting this in perspective, 97 percent of that water is saline or salt water in the oceans, and only 3 percent is fresh water. Of this 3 percent fresh water, 68.7 percent is found in ice caps and glaciers; 30.1 percent is considered ground water, with only 0.3 percent of this fresh water being found on the surface. Of the 0.3 percent on the surface, 87 percent is found in lakes, 11 percent in swamps, and 2 percent in rivers. So we should recognize how little of earth's water is usable by humans. Of all the water on the earth, only 3 percent is usable and the vast majority of that is relatively inaccessible, either locked in ice caps and glaciers or found underground. A very small percentage is actually easily available on the surface.

Water's physical and chemical characteristics are extremely important when we consider that life is not possible without its presence. The water molecule is H_2O, or two hydrogen atoms that are covalently bound to one oxygen atom. Water is a polar molecule because oxygen has greater electronegativity than does hydrogen, which means that the oxygen atom attracts more electrons than the two hydrogen atoms do. Because of the higher electronegativity of the oxygen atom, the water molecule acts like a molecular polar magnet with a negative pole at the oxygen molecule and a positive pole with the two hydrogen atoms. For this reason water, which is a polar solvent, becomes a universal solvent in that all dissolvable substances other than nonpolar substances, such as fats, will dissolve in water. In addition, because of this polarity, water molecules are very cohesive in their liquid state. This is a critical physical property, because when water freezes, the water molecules become slightly more separated, and solid water, or ice, is less dense than liquid water and therefore floats in water. This is a characteristic shared by very few substances and is vital to the development and maintenance of life. We have all heard the term "you only see the tip of the iceberg." This refers to the fact that ice is less dense than water and even though 90 percent of a floating piece of ice is below the surface, the fact is that ice floats in liquid water. This is important not just for recreational activities. If solid water, or ice, were more dense than the liquid water, which is true of most other substances, lakes, rivers and streams, and the ocean would freeze from the bottom up. If that occurred, the seasons as we experience them on this planet would never create a summer season long enough or warm enough to fully thaw the massive bodies of water on our planet. Just the most superficial surface area would thaw and the earth would be a solid globe of ice (and would act as a planet-sized heat sink). Obviously, life as we know it could neither develop nor be maintained in such an environment, so the fact that ice is less dense than water is a critical factor in the development and maintenance of life.

Those of us in developed nations really do not worry about where we get our water. We are used to free, safe water coming from the tap and have now developed the expectation that we will be able to buy purified water wherever we go. This is not true in the developing world.

According to the WHO, 2 percent of the world's population does not have access to safe drinking water and frequently have to travel substantial distances to obtain it. This task most often falls to women. They at times have to walk five to ten miles a day roundtrip and generally try to carry between five and ten gallons of water on their trip back from the source. Water weighs 8.3 pounds per gallon, so they can be carrying between forty and eighty pounds on their heads.

In addition, this is frequently water of questionable quality that we would be extremely reluctant to bathe in, much less drink.

SANITATION

In the United States, we are used to clean sanitation facilities, and toilets can actually become designer items in our homes. Compare this to 40 percent of the world's population that does not have access to even the most basic sanitation facilities.

It is for these reasons that the Millennium Development Project has chosen as the seventh goal the ensuring of environmental sustainability, with target 10 being to halve by 2015 the proportion of people without sustainable access to safe drinking water and basic sanitation.

The basic demographics of lack of access to safe drinking water or adequate sanitation are appalling, as noted above: 20 percent of the world's population, or 1.3 billion people, have no safe source of drinking water. Double that, 40 percent of the world's population, or 2.6 billion people, have no choice but to defecate in buckets, plastic bags or open fields every day and do not even have access to a pit latrine. [10]

The world saw the effects of this in Haiti in October 2010, when during the flooding season the fields and living areas were flooded by the Artibonite River. Of course, the fields were being used for sanitation, and when they flooded the sanitation areas were in direct contact with the river and other water supplies. Not long thereafter, the cholera epidemic began. At latest count there have been more than 500,000 cases and 7,000 deaths. It must be noted that until relief efforts for the 2010 earthquake, cholera had not been seen in the Caribbean since the mid-nineteenth century, and the evidence shows that the organism was brought to Haiti from outside sources since the strain is most genetically related to organisms isolated in Bangladesh. [11]

The lack of access to basic sanitation and safe water is responsible for the death of 3,900 children each day, or 1.4 million a year. This robs the poor, especially women and children, of their time, health, and dignity and thwarts progress toward all the Millennium Development goals, especially in Africa and Asia. [10] As noted by the Millennium Development report, diseases transmitted through water or human excrement are the second leading cause of death among children worldwide after respiratory disease. Far more people suffer the ill effects of poor water supply and sanitation than are affected by war and terrorism, and one has to ask, is there a link between people's lack of access to basic human needs and the proliferation of war and terrorism in the world?

In 2002, the United Nations affirmed the right to water, noting that such a right is indispensable for leading a life of human dignity and a prerequisite for the realization of the other human rights. In 2003, the UN proclaimed 2005–2015 the international decade for action. Water is life: "water is critical for sustainable development including environmental integrity and the eradication of poverty and hunger and is indispensable for human health and wellbeing."

Water is essential for well-being and a basic requirement for the healthy functioning of all ecosystems. A combination of safe drinking water, adequate sanitation, and hygienic practices such as hand washing is recognized as a precondition for reducing morbidity and mortality rates, especially among children. Sufficient water for washing and safe, private sanitation facilities are central to the basic rights of every human being for personal dignity and self-respect. [10]

We should reiterate in this section some of the water-related diseases that are the most common causes of illness and death among the poor in developing countries, responsible for 1.6 million deaths a year. These include the diarrheal diseases carried both by viruses as well as bacteria; helminthic or worm infestation such as ascariasis; hookworm, which in parts of the world is the major cause of iron deficiency anemia; dracunculiasis as discussed in a previous section; schistosomiasis; and trachoma. Of note, cholera, typhoid fever, dysentery, and polio are all transmitted by fecal-oral spread, in large part by contaminated water supplies due to inadequate sanitation and lack of access to potable water.

SUMMARY

In the first part of this chapter we reviewed the basics of nutrition and defined protein-energy malnutrition and kwashiorkor. We discussed the epidemiology and metrics used to evaluate individuals who are malnourished and therefore susceptible to disease because of a compromised immune system. We have talked about a few of the historical epidemic diseases associated with famine, in part to reiterate some of the principles we discussed in earlier chapters and in part to set the stage for the more contemporary plagues.

The interaction between microbes and their hosts is complex, involving microbial factors such as virulence and the life cycle of the organism, and host factors including habits, hygiene, and possible compromise of natural defenses. In each case, we see that improved nutrition and preventive public health measures, such as improved sanitation and protection of the water supply, far outweigh medical therapy in terms of potential lives saved.

REFERENCES

1. Sachs J. The end of poverty. New York: Penguin Books, 2006.
2. Food and Agriculture Organization of the United Nations website, http://www.fao.org/publications/SOFI/en/, accessed January 2, 2014.
3. United States Department of Agriculture website, www.ers.usda.gov/publications/erreconomic-researchreport/err-155.aspx, accessed on January 2, 2014.

4. World Health Organization website, http://www.who.int/nutri tion/topics/vad/en/, accessed on January 2, 2014.

5. Black RE, Morris SS, Bryce J. Where and why are 10 million children dying every year? *Lancet.* 2003 Jun 28;361(9376):2226–34.

6. Kotloff KL, Winickoff JP, Ivanoff B, Clemens JD, Swerdlow DL, Sansonetti PJ, et al. Global burden of Shigella infections: Implications for vaccine development and implementation of control strategies. Bull WHO. 1999; 77: 651–666.

7. Mandell, Bennett, Dolin. Principles & practice of infectious diseases, 6th ed. Philadelphia: Elsevier, 2005: 2657–2659.

8. Gunnlaugsson G. et al. Funerals during the 1994 cholera epidemic in Guinea-Bissau, West Africa: The need for disinfection of bodies of persons dying of cholera. *Epidemiol Infect.* 1998; 120:7.

9. Crump JA, Luby SP, Mintz ED. The global burden of typhoid fever. Bull WHO May 2004, 82 (5).

10. U.N. Millennium Project Task Force on Water—Health, dignity and development: what will it take?

11. Ali A, Chen Y, Johnson JA, Redden E, Mayette Y, Rashid MH, et al. Recent clonal origin of cholera in Haiti. *Emerg Infect Dis.* Apr 2011; 17(4): 699–701.

7

LOUD EMERGENCIES I
HIV/AIDS

Lisa V. Adams

THE DAWN OF AN EPIDEMIC

In Chapter 4, you read the brief case of a patient who presented in an urban emergency room with an unknown respiratory illness and severe immune suppression in 1978. It wasn't until 1981 that the first report of unusual pneumonias and oral yeast infections in four previously healthy gay men was published in the *New England Journal of Medicine.* [1] It would be another three years before the first report of human immunodeficiency virus (HIV)/acquired immunodeficiency syndrome (AIDS) in Africa, from the Democratic Republic of Congo, then Zaire, was published. [2] These thirty-eight patients, of whom half were women, did not have any of the risk factors of homosexual sex, intravenous drug use, or blood transfusions seen in the U.S. patients. The authors concluded that AIDS in Africa seemed to present a new epidemiologic setting for AIDS, one in which heterosexual sex is the main mode of transmission.

Today, it is estimated that there are between 34.2 and 38.8 million people living with HIV. [3] Two important metrics—new infections and AIDS deaths—have been decreasing over the past few years; in 2012, there were estimated to be between 1.9 and 2.7 million new HIV infections and between 1.4 and 1.9 million AIDS deaths. [3]

With growing populations in the large urban centers of most

African countries in the 1980s and 1990s, the setting was ripe for the spread of HIV. By 1985, one seroprevalence survey showed that 56 percent of a group of ninety commercial sex workers in Nairobi had antibodies to HIV (indicating infection); this rate jumped to 66 percent when evaluated in commercial sex workers of lower socioeconomic status. [4] In the late 1990s, data also emerged demonstrating the relationship between a history of other sexually transmitted diseases, especially those causing genital ulcers, and HIV infection. [5] Higher HIV rates were also observed in uncircumcised men, which eventually led to the wide-scale circumcision programs in Africa as a preventive measure. [6] Studies of discordant couples—where one partner is HIV-infected and the other is not—also showed viral load to be the strongest predictor of HIV transmission. [6] This information and further studies that demonstrated reduced transmission with effective antiretroviral treatment led to the game-changing concept of "treatment as prevention." [7]

ORIGIN OF THE VIRUS

HIV is a zoonosis. The human immunodeficiency virus is closely related to the primate virus simian immunodeficiency virus (SIV). In fact, the SIV that infects chimpanzees is virtually identical to human HIV-1. [8] In the early 1900s, SIV was transmitted sporadically to humans in Central Africa primarily through practices related to skinning and preparing bush meat or eating uncooked meat. Molecular clock analysis—a technique based on the relatively constant mutation rate associated with evolution and used to estimate the timing of biological events—of diverse strains of HIV suggests that the most recent common ancestor of HIV-1 jumped species from chimps to humans in approximately 1921. The implicated chimpanzee species only lives north and west of the Congo River, which may have helped contain spread of the virus. It is speculated that there were sporadic unrecognized human cases in rural areas in western and west-central Africa without significant spread for decades. Later we will see how that pattern changed and resulted in a major pandemic, with the earliest epicenter of human cases being Kinshasa, the capital of the Democratic Republic of Congo.

In 1984, the virus was isolated and named HIV-I. It was in 1985 that the first diagnostic test was approved; this test relied on the detection of antibodies to the virus to make the diagnosis. It would be another two years before the first drug—zidovudine, known more commonly as AZT—would be approved for the treatment of HIV. The triumph of the first AIDS drug was short-lived, as its efficacy was not permanent, presumably due to the rapid development of resistance with a single-drug regimen. It would be another ten years, in 1996, when the development of the newest class of drugs, protease inhibitors, would change the treatment landscape. With their introduction and effect on blocking viral replication, for the first time since the recognition of HIV in the United States, mortality from the disease began to decline.

MODES OF TRANSMISSION AND PATHOGENESIS

HIV can be transmitted by one of three means: (1) through sexual contact, (2) parenterally (e.g., through the use of unclean needles or receiving a transfusion of contaminated blood products), or (3) from mother to child, either during pregnancy, at the time of birth, or through breastfeeding. In high-income countries, HIV transmission is more commonly via homosexual rather than heterosexual sex, and through intravenous drug use. In low-income countries, HIV transmission occurs more often through heterosexual sex and through the use of unsterile needles or unsafe transfusions (though the latter practices are now fortunately less common). HIV transmission through sexual contact is bidirectional, and the risk is approximately ten times as high early in infection when the viral load is often highest and the infected person may not yet be aware that he or she is infected. Transmission from a contaminated needle is particularly effective. The risk from each exposure is approximately 1 percent, which is about 10 times the risk associated with sexual transmission.

Most perinatal transmission from mother to child occurs during labor and delivery (where there is frequent exposure to maternal blood) or during breastfeeding, which traditionally would be done for more than a year or often until the birth of the next child. A focus on preventing mother-to-child transmission (PMTCT programs) has been a major focus of HIV prevention activities. In 1994, results were announced by the AIDS Clinical Trials Group from the first successful PMTCT interventional study that administering AZT to pregnant women during pregnancy and labor and then to their newborns for the first six weeks reduced the risk of HIV transmission by approximately two-thirds. [9] In subsequent years a much simpler regimen—referred to as single-dose neviripine since it involved administering a single dose of the antiretroviral medication neviripine to the woman during labor and a single dose to the infant after birth—became a widespread intervention in resource-limited settings. Current recommendations are for pregnant women to receive combination antiretroviral therapy (not just a single drug), the most effective measure for reducing mother-to-child transmission. Avoiding breastfeeding and exclusively bottle feeding is the safest option in terms of HIV risk, but in settings where that is not feasible (due to cultural acceptability, cost, and lack of clean water for formula preparation), the World Health Organization (WHO) recommends exclusive breastfeeding for the first six months of life with rapid weaning. Breast milk is the best nutritional option for an infant and has been shown to confer various health benefits, so the option of six months of breastfeeding provides the most important benefits of breast milk to the infant.

Once a person is infected, the virus attacks the cells of the immune system, specifically CD4 lymphocytes. These important immune defense cells are so named for the CD4 protein that lines their surface and to which HIV attaches. CD4 cells are important actors in the host immune response as they stimulate B cells to produce antibodies and help to regulate other cells in eliminating other infectious agents. Like all viruses, HIV will first bind to, then enter its target cell and take over the cell's internal machinery to replicate itself. HIV, however, is a retrovirus, which means that it integrates its genetic material into that of the host cell's, thereby establishing a permanent infection. Eventually, the virus destroys the CD4 cell. Over time, the virus will deplete the body of these important defender cells, leaving the body susceptible to all kinds of opportunistic infections, so called because they can only thrive when the opportunity of a suppressed immune system is present. If left untreated, most people will eventually die from one or more of these infections.

HOW HIV SPREAD IN AFRICA

Given the evidence that the first transmission of chimpanzee SIV from animal to human occurred around 1920, why did HIV not become widespread at that time? What factors contributed to the spread of HIV in the decades that followed?

In his book *The Origin of AIDS*, Jacques Pepin describes his well-researched and highly plausible explanation of the circumstances that led to widespread transmission of HIV in Africa. [10] He outlines the factors present in the1960s and 1970s that led to the first cases of AIDS being diagnosed in the United States in 1981 and a few years later in Africa. Dr. Pepin, an infectious disease specialist who worked in Zaire (now the Democratic Republic of Congo) as a medical officer in the 1980s, applies epidemiology principles to the bushmeat origin theory of HIV to explain how the virus could spread from one bush hunter in Central Africa to so many others. He describes the large-scale medical campaigns implemented by Belgian and French colonists in the 1940s through the 1960s that led to thousands of West Africans receiving injections for a variety of infectious diseases including African sleeping sickness, malaria, and leprosy. The problem was that the needle sterilization practices were inadequate, resulting in the perfect setup for transmission of a blood-borne pathogen such as HIV. This means of widespread transmission was further fueled by the concurrent factors of urbanization and social unrest in places such as Kinshasa at that time, which was accompanied by increases in commercial sex. Dissemination to other areas, including the United States, likely occurred through travel and subsequent sexual transmission. Spread of the virus to Haiti is speculated to have resulted from transmission to the Haitians hired by the UN to work as administrators and teachers in Africa once the French-speaking Belgians left the region. It is estimated some that four thousand Haitians were hired in the 1960s to work in Africa.

While there have been a few other theories to describe the origin of HIV and its widespread dissemination, Dr. Pepin's theory is currently at the forefront. Epidemiologic modeling has shown that HIV could not have spread as widely as it did solely through sexual transmission. It is tragic and ironic that programs to eradicate tropical diseases (even if the colonists were the main intended beneficiary) could have contributed to one of the worst pandemics in our recent history.

INTRODUCING ANTIRETROVIRAL MEDICATIONS IN AFRICA: THE FIGHT FOR ACCESS

The first breakthroughs in antiretroviral drug discovery were critical to changing the course of the HIV pandemic. Following the introduction of protease inhibitors in 1996, combination therapy became the mainstay of HIV treatment in the United States. In the subsequent years, antitretroviral therapy (ART) was limited to those living in high-income countries, or the few wealthy individuals living in middle- and low-income countries. Cost was the predominant barrier, since all medications were still under patent and prohibitively expensive. The Agreement on Trade Related Aspects of Intellectual Property Rights (known as the TRIPS agreement) introduced intellectual property law into the international trading system and seemed to be a means of ensuring that no affordable generic ART medications would be developed while patents were still active. Discussions in the United States were limited about whether ART could be introduced in low-income countries, settings where households and communities were being devastated by the loss of their young parents and main income earners in the peak of their economically productive years. When pressed, most involved in the discourse cited the numerous challenges associated with ART rollout in such a setting. In addition to cost, the lack of trained health care workers in ART administration and management, the lack of infrastructure to distribute medications, and the need to tightly control use were often raised as principle obstacles to increased ART access. In 2001, a leading U.S. administrator commented on the challenge of having to take these drugs on a strict schedule and that "many Africans don't know what Western time is." [11] Sadly, there appeared a general resignation to one more global health inequity framed by a person's (or country's) inability to pay.

In 2001, the ART access debate began to heat up on the international stage. World health officials, patients, and patient advocates began to call for action. A group of Yale students together with representatives from Doctors Without Borders (the U.S. branch of the nongovernmental medical relief organization Médecins Sans Frontières) brought pressure on Yale and a pharmaceutical manufacturer to allow South Africa to import a generic form of one antiretroviral medication, stavudine. In 1998, thirty-nine drug makers had sued the South African government over its claimed right to purchase lower-cost ART medications. In April 2001, the pharmaceutical companies dropped the case, conceding that the South African law permitting the government to purchase brand-name drugs at the lowest rates available was in compliance with international trade agreements. One of the largest generic manufacturers in India sought permission to sell its products to low-income countries; costs of medications fell from $10,000 to about $600 per patient per year. In November 2001, the Doha Declaration on the TRIPS Agreement was adopted; this statement re-affirmed the flexibility of the TRIPS Agreement to allow access to essential medications. As U.S. pharmaceutical companies began selling their antiretroviral medications at cost over the next years, this became the norm. Interestingly, increasing access to ART medications did not cause the collapse of the pharmaceutical industry, and to everyone's benefit, drug research and innovation continue to thrive.

Today it is unimaginable to think of high-prevalent HIV settings in Africa and elsewhere without access to ART. The focus now is on universal access. While country responses have varied to some extent, several African countries such as Botswana and Rwanda have been at the forefront of the universal access campaign and today report more than 80 percent of their eligible HIV-infected patients are receiving these life-saving medicines. Other important prevention measures such as screening of the blood supply and distributing condoms are also widespread in most high-prevalent settings. And the concern about whether non-Westerners could adhere to complicated ART regimens? As early as 2003, when ART regimens were still fairly complex, the data showed that Africans actually had very high rates of treatment adherence, achieving 90 percent adherence, considerably higher than the average of 70 percent adherence among Americans. [12]

PREVENTING HIV

Preventing new HIV infections is essential to controlling the epidemic. Short of the development of an effective vaccine, it does not appear that there is a single prevention intervention or strategy that will be applicable in all settings. Instead, a menu of prevention options is needed for different settings based on the disease epidemiology and target population(s). Depending on whether the epidemic is generalized (i.e., greater than 1 percent of the general population is infected) or targeted (i.e., present primarily in certain high-risk groups), different strategies may be indicated. In the early days of the epidemic, the "ABC" approach, an acronym for "Abstinence, Be faithful, use Condoms," was promoted. Aside from the controversy over whether abstinence should be the only option offered to unmarried youth, it is clear that all three recommendations formed the foundation of prevention activities. These three approaches, however, were not enough. While promoting abstinence among youth tended to delay the age of sexual debut, this also only delayed, rather than prevented, acquisition of HIV. Being faithful while married requires adherence by both partners, and many monogamous married women have found themselves contacting HIV from their nonmonogamous husbands. For condoms to reach their maximal protective effect of 80 to 90 percent, they must be used correctly and consistently. Development of the female condom was an effort to place a prevention option in the hands of the woman, but their use still requires some male partner acceptance. For unclear reasons, female condoms do not appear to be as widely used or available as male condoms. Microbicides were another hoped for preventive technique that could be female-controlled, but effectiveness has not achieved even 50 percent.

It should be noted that all of the above interventions require changes in behavior. While there is no doubt that many people across the globe have made significant adjustments in their behavior because of the HIV epidemic, individual-level behavior change can be challenging to maintain, especially once the epidemic is under some control and the threat of risk is less or is less apparent.

Male circumcision is another means of preventing HIV transmission. Randomized controlled trials performed in eastern and southern Africa have demonstrated a roughly 60 percent reduction in heterosexually acquired HIV among men who were circumcised. [13] Furthermore, this benefit appears to be sustained for approximately six years following the procedure. [13] In 2007, the WHO and the Joint United Nations Programme on HIV/AIDS (UNAIDS) recommended voluntary medical male circumcision be promoted as an HIV prevention measure in fourteen African countries with a generalized HIV epidemic and low rates of male circumcision. To date, millions of male circumcisions have been performed for HIV prevention purposes. Given the relationship described above between other sexually transmitted diseases (STDs) and HIV transmission, prompt diagnosis and treatment of STDs has been promoted as another means of controlling HIV.

In settings where use of contaminated needles is a main mode of HIV transmission, needle exchange programs have proven effective. These sometimes controversial "harm reduction" programs provide sterile needles in exchange for used needles, with the premise being that is it better to reduce the harm incurred from unchecked HIV transmission than from illegal drug use.

In 2011, the results of a landmark study were released that demonstrated a 96 percent protective effect among couples in which one partner was HIV-infected and the other was not. [14] This randomized, controlled trial, which showed that transmission was significantly reduced by reducing the viral load in the infected person's blood, heralded a new era in HIV treatment and prevention with the new emphasis of "treatment as prevention." With increasing availability of more effective and better-tolerated antiretroviral medications, treatment initiation has been shifting to earlier in the course of disease. When there were fewer drug choices, the treatment approach was to wait and "reserve" medication use until the time when viral replication increased and the viral load began to rise. Having a variety of different drug classes (which have different mechanisms of action) and more effective drugs that are better tolerated provides more options for patients who may develop intolerable side effects with a particular medication or have a resistant strain. Today, a person in the United States may be started on medications once diagnosed with HIV infection. Most patients should be able to have their viral load maintained at an undetectable level with a simple once or twice daily regimen of medicines that do not cause undesirable side effects.

Elsewhere in the world, many low-income countries, where the drug choices are more limited, are adopting the WHO guidelines, which recommend starting patients on medications when their CD4 falls below 500 (much higher than the recent threshold of 350 or the original threshold of 200) or they reach a specific clinical stage of their disease. We can expect most countries to move toward an earlier start of antiretroviral medications for all their HIV-infected patients in the future as their resources allow. All HIV-infected patients who are diagnosed with TB are eligible to start antiretrovirals regardless of their CD4 count. Similarly, the WHO now recommends all HIV-infected pregnant or breast-feeding women be started on triple-drug ART regardless of CD4 count or clinical stage; where possible, treatment is continued for life (previously referred to as "option B+"). [15] Their infants receive a course of medication based on the drug regimen that the mother is taking for a duration determined by whether the infant is breastfeeding or not. Lastly, oral pre-exposure prophylaxis of HIV (PrEP)—which is the daily use of antiretroviral drugs by an non-HIV-infected individual to block the acquisition of HIV—has been shown to be effective in certain circumstances, namely, in sero-discordant couples and people who inject drugs [15]. This option may be an additional intervention for the uninfected partner or individual at risk.

Research to develop an HIV vaccine is ongoing. Development of a single vaccine has been hampered by both the virus's ability to mutate rapidly to evade immune responses and the range of immunologically different virus subtypes that vary by region. Furthermore, unlike other viruses, only a minority of those infected with HIV produce the broadly neutralizing antibodies that are considered the gold standard for effective viral vaccine development. These antibodies are most useful because they provide protection against a variety of pathogenic strains.

After decades of failed attempts to induce either protective antibody responses or T-cell control of viral replication, an unexpected success was reported in 2009 from Thailand. The Thai Phase III vaccine trial (known as RV144) tested a combination of two vaccines, the ALVAC® HIV vaccine and the AIDSVAX® B/E vaccine. [16] Given in succession, these vaccines work as a prime-boost combination, with the doses of the first vaccine, ALVAC® HIV, priming the immune system and the doses of the second vaccine, AIDSVAX® B/E, boosting the response. The RV144 trial enrolled more than sixteen thousand volunteers. In addition to demonstrating safety and tolerability, the researchers found that the use of the two candidate vaccine series lowered the rate of HIV infection by 31 percent in the intervention group compared to the placebo-receiving control group. While this modest level of protection was not enough to warrant regulatory approval of the vaccines, this trial has provided useful information that is being used to inform further vaccine development and lead to new studies of booster vaccine doses. Recently published findings from the extensive RV144 laboratory data are helping researchers better understand the protective immune responses, which may help them prioritize vaccine candidates for future clinical trials and accelerate the overall process of HIV vaccine development. [17] Several additional vaccine candidates are currently under clinical investigation, mostly in the early phases of study. A myriad of collaborators are involved in HIV vaccine research, including the U.S. Military HIV Research Program, the U.S. Centers for Disease Control and Prevention, the Center for HIV/AIDS Vaccine Immunology (CHAVI), the HIV Vaccine Trials Network, the Collaboration for AIDS Vaccine Discovery, and multiple university partners.

CONCLUSION

HIV has impacted global health in many significant ways. Historians have referred to our handling of the most vulnerable in society as a measure of our humanity. How we have responded to the HIV pandemic may be one of those important gauges of our sense of human rights and humanity used by those that come after us. The progress made in addressing this pandemic in the arenas of diagnostics, drug discovery, access to care, and public health has been formidable, and it has influenced research and practices in these areas related to all infectious diseases. Some refer to how HIV succeeded in reshaping global health. The aim of this chapter has been to discuss some of the social aspects of the HIV pandemic with an appreciation for how far-reaching and pivotal it has been in our recent history.

REFERENCES

1. Gottlieb MS, Schroff R, Schanker HM, Weisman JD, Fan PT, Wolf RA, et al. Pneumocystis carinii pneumonia and mucosal candidiasis in previously healthy homosexual men: evidence of a new acquired cellular immunodeficiency. *N Engl J Med*. 1981 Dec 10;305(24):1425–31.

2. Piot P, Quinn TC, Taelman H, Feinsod FM, Minlangu KB, Wobin O, et al. Acquired immunodeficiency syndrome in a heterosexual population in Zaire. *Lancet*. 1984 Jul 14;2(8394):65–9.

3. UNAIDS. Global report: UNAIDS report on the global AIDS epidemic 2013. UNAIDS / JC2502/1/E.

4. Kreiss JK, Koech D, Plummer FA, Holmes KK, Lightfoote M, Piot P, et al. AIDS virus infection in Nairobi prostitutes. Spread of the epidemic to East Africa. *N Engl J Med*. 1986 Feb 13;314(7):414–8.

5. Simonsen JN, Cameron DW, Gakinya MN, Ndinya-Achola JO, D'Costa LJ, Karasira P, et al. Human immunodeficiency virus infection among men with sexually transmitted diseases. Experience from a center in Africa. *N Engl J Med*. 1988 Aug 4;319(5):274–8.

6. Quinn TC, Wawer MJ, Sewankambo N, Serwadda D, Li C, Wabwire-Mangen F, et al. Viral load and heterosexual transmission of human immunodeficiency virus type 1. Rakai Project Study Group. *N Engl J Med*. 2000 Mar 30;342(13):921–9.

7. Cohen MS, Chen YQ, McCauley M, Gamble T, Hosseinipour MC, Kumarasamy N, et al.; HPTN 052 Study Team. Prevention of HIV-1 infection with early antiretroviral therapy. *N Engl J Med*. 2011 Aug 11;365(6):493–505.

8. Hahn BH, Shaw GM, De Cock KM, Sharp PM. AIDS as a zoonosis: scientific and public health implications. *Science*. 2000 Jan 28;287(5453):607–14.

9. Connor EM, Sperling RS, Gelber R, Kiselev P, Scott G, O'Sullivan MJ, et al. Reduction of maternal-infant transmission of human immunodeficiency virus type 1 with zidovudine treatment. Pediatric AIDS Clinical Trials Group Protocol 076 Study Group. *N Engl J Med*. 1994 Nov 3;331(18):1173–80.

10. Pepin J. The origin of AIDS. New York: Cambridge University Press, 2011.

11. Donnelly J. Prevention urged in AIDS fight: Natsios says fund

LOUD EMERGENCIES, HIV/AIDS

should spend less on HIV treatment. *The Boston Globe,* 2001 June 7; Sect A:8.

12. McNeil DG Jr. Africans outdo U.S. patients in following AIDS therapy. *New York Times,* 2003 September 3. http://www.nytimes.com/2003/09/03/world/africans-outdo-us-patients-in-following-aids-therapy.html?pagewanted=all&src=pm.

13. Centers for Disease Control and Prevention (CDC). Voluntary medical male circumcision—southern and eastern Africa, 2010–2012. *Morb Mortal Wkly Rep.* 2013 Nov 29;62(47):953–7.

14. Cohen M, Chen YQ, McCauley M, Gamble T, Hosseinipour MC, Kumarasamy N, et al. Prevention of HIV-1 infection with early antiretroviral therapy. *N Engl J Med.* 2011;365(6):493–505.

15. World Health Organization. Consolidated guidelines on the use of antiretroviral drugs for treating and preventing HIV infection: recommendations for a public health approach. Geneva: World Health Organization, June 2013. http://apps.who.int/iris/bitstream/10665/85321/1/9789241505727_eng.pdf, accessed June 15, 2014.

16. Rerks-Ngarm S, Pitisuttithum P, Nitayaphan S, Kaewkungwal J, Chiu J, Paris R; MOPH-TAVEG Investigators. Vaccination with ALVAC and AIDSVAX to prevent HIV-1 infection in Thailand. *N Engl J Med.* 2009 Dec 3;361(23):2209–20.

17. Haynes BF, Gilbert PB, McElrath MJ, Zolla-Pazner S, Tomaras GD, Alam SM, et al. Immune-correlates analysis of an HIV-1 vaccine efficacy trial. *N Engl J Med.* 2012 Apr 5;366(14):1275–86.

8

LOUD EMERGENCIES II

Tuberculosis

Lisa V. Adams

AN ANCIENT DISEASE

Tuberculosis is considered an ancient disease that has afflicted humans throughout the centuries. Known in the vernacular as "consumption" because the disease appears to consume its sufferer from within, tuberculosis classically presents as a person who is very thin, pale, feverish, and has an unrelenting cough that produces bloody sputum. During the Romance era, many an artist, writer, or musician had tuberculosis; it was so common among these groups that for a period it seemed tuberculosis was linked to artistic talent. Some considered it the price artists paid for their gifts. Elizabeth Barrett Browning apparently quoted a contemporary who wondered, "is it possible that genius is only scrofula?" [1] (scrofula is a name for tuberculosis in the lymph nodes). Others saw the connection resulting from the apparent freeing of the mind and creative abilities as the physical body was consumed or became wasted by the disease. From the Bronte sisters to Chopin to Voltaire, the long list of acclaimed poets, writers, artists, politicians, and musicians to have suffered from or lost their lives to tuberculosis indicates how prevalent the disease was in the era before effective treatment was available.

TUBERCULOSIS: THE BASICS

Tuberculosis is caused by the bacteria *Mycobacterium tuberculosis* (MTB). An "oxygen-seeking" organism, it grows most successfully in tissues with a high oxygen content such as the apices of the human lung. It is primarily an intracellular pathogen, usually infecting cells of the immune system, which helps it hide from the body's defenses. It is a slow-growing bacteria (compare its generation time of twelve to eighteen hours to that of twenty to thirty minutes for another common human bacterial pathogen, E. coli), which makes it a challenge to grow in culture media. Rather than having a culture result in two to three days, it can take two to twelve weeks for MTB to grow; this long lag time greatly decreases the utility of culture results in managing individual patients.

The high lipid content in the MTB cell wall makes the bacteria impermeable to the usual stains used to identify organisms (e.g., the Gram stain) so special reagents are used to detect MTB. The MTB bacteria are known as "acid-fast bacilli" because of their staining characteristics in the laboratory, and the slide that is prepared using a specimen from a presumptive TB patient is referred to as an AFB smear. Tuberculosis can affect almost any organ of the body, but most cases are pulmonary (80 percent of all tuberculosis cases worldwide) followed by tuberculosis of the lymph nodes (tuberculosis lymphadenitis) and the bones (osteoarticular tuberculosis, also known as Potts Disease when it affects the spine). A patient with tuberculosis in an extrapulmonary site will present with symptoms based on the site affected, usually with pain and swelling at the main site of infection.

Tuberculosis is spread through airborne transmission. When a person with pulmonary tuberculosis coughs, sneezes, sings, or laughs, small respiratory droplets are aerosolized and released into the airspace. These infectious droplet nuclei may only contain a few MTB bacilli, but a person needs to inhale only a few to become infected. Droplet nuclei have been found to linger in the air for up to eight hours. Sunlight (UV rays) kills MTB and good ventilation ensures the droplet nuclei are dispersed (and ideally carried outside). Given these transmission dynamics, it is clear why dark, overcrowded, and poorly ventilated living quarters create the perfect environment for tuberculosis transmission. One untreated person with pulmonary tuberculosis will infect an average of ten to fifteen people in a year.

Once the MTB bacilli are inhaled, their small size helps them evade the mucociliary defenses of the bronchial tree so they are deposited in the terminal airspaces of the lung. The tuberculosis bacilli then have four potential fates: (1) they may be killed by the immune system, (2) they may multiply and cause disease (this is also called primary TB), (3) they may become dormant and remain dormant for life (latent TB infection), or (4) they may become dormant and later in life reactivate to cause disease (reactivation disease). The health of the infected person largely determines which of these outcomes occurs. Only 10 percent of immunocompetent people (those with healthy immune systems) infected with MTB will develop tuberculosis disease in their lifetime; the remaining 90 percent never become ill (and therefore cannot transmit the organism). Among those with a compromised immune system (e.g., those with HIV infection or malnutrition) or immature immune systems (e.g., infants), the proportion that develops TB disease is much higher. In those with HIV infection—the greatest risk factor for progressing from latent TB infection to TB disease—the risk jumps from a 10 percent *lifetime* risk to a 10 percent *annual* risk. Tuberculosis has a high mortality rate if untreated. Natural history data from the pre-chemotherapy era tell us that by the end of five years, 50 percent of untreated pulmonary TB patients will have died, 25 percent will have self-cured, and the remaining 25 percent will have a chronic form of infectious tuberculosis.

TUBERCULOSIS EPIDEMIOLOGY AND CONTROL

While tuberculosis is present in every region of the globe, control efforts have focused on the twenty-two highest-burden countries. These countries are home to 80 percent of the world's TB patients. This ranking is based on absolute numbers and not rates, therefore, India and China are—and will likely remain—at the top of the list. The overarching goal of tuberculosis control worldwide is, quite simply, to reduce morbidity and mortality from tuberculosis. This can only be achieved by decreasing disease transmission, which requires preventing transmission from an infectious tuberculosis patient to a contact. To prevent transmission, cases must be identified as early as possible and standardized treatment begun promptly to promote swift sputum conversion from positive AFB smears to negative ones (a measure of infectiousness) and to prevent the emergence of drug resistance. Infection prevention techniques, such as good cough etiquette (e.g., coughing into tissues, your elbow, or your handkerchief) and ensuring adequate air ventilation are things that can be done in any setting and are actively being promoted in most low-income countries (LICs). Tracing of contacts—to identify secondary cases and those with latent TB infection—is limited to identifying household contacts, especially children under age five and any immunosuppressed individuals, and asking them to come to the clinic for evaluation. Preventing the development of drug resistance is critical to effective TB control. If we lose the battle to drug resistance, all of the hard-won gains we have made over the last several decades will be lost.

In 1991, the 44th World Health Assembly set TB control targets to be achieved by the year 2000, but in view of the slow progress being made in many high-burden countries, the target date was postponed to 2005. These global targets were (1) to successfully treat 85 percent of detected smear-positive TB cases and (2) to detect at least 70 percent of estimated smear-positive cases. Modeling and epidemiological analysis tells us that if these two goals are achieved, both TB prevalence and the rate of TB transmission will decrease immediately. TB incidence will begin to decrease gradually, and there will be little acquired drug resistance. An important caveat is that these models were applied to low-HIV-prevalence settings, so the same benefits may not be seen in high-HIV-prevalence settings. The second goal of detecting at least 70 percent of the estimated sputum smear-positive cases will ensure that most cases are identified and will not remain untreated in the community. Case detection efforts should only be intensified, however, once a high cure rate is achieved. Otherwise, there is a risk of overwhelming the diagnostic and treatment services with excess cases that a TB program and its health care delivery system cannot manage, resulting in incomplete care, poor outcomes, and the potential for emerging drug resistance.

Case detection rate is determined by dividing the number of newly notified cases countrywide by the estimated incidence for the country. This requires having estimates of the TB incidence for each country in the world. TB incidence is never directly measured at the national level; to do so would require following the population (or at least large cohorts) for a long time, which would be costly and impractical. In countries with a high burden of TB, prevalence can be directly measured through nationwide surveys, using sample sizes of forty to fifty thousand people, with costs in the range of $1 million or more per survey.

Until recently, estimates of incidence were based on the 1997 figures that were meticulously calculated by the WHO surveillance division and adjusted yearly based on many smaller surveys. Between 2009 and 2011, consultations with ninety-six countries that account for about 90 percent of the world's TB cases were conducted, and these led to a major updating of estimates of TB incidence, mortality, and prevalence, particularly for countries in the African region. The case detection rate is a measure of a na-

---

BOX 8-1

THE DOTS STRATEGY

The five components of the DOTS strategy are as follows:

1. Sustained political commitment
2. Case detection by quality-assured sputum smear microscopy
3. Treatment of TB cases with standard short-course chemotherapy regimens under proper case-management conditions, including direct observation of treatment
4. Uninterrupted supply of quality-assured anti-TB drugs
5. Recording and reporting system enabling outcome assessment and management of program effectiveness

---

tional TB program's ability to diagnose and collect data on TB cases. High detection rates mean that transmission by undiagnosed cases is curtailed and will lead to less TB disease and fewer TB deaths in the population.

THE DOTS STRATEGY:
A COMPREHENSIVE PACKAGE FOR TB CONTROL

Through the brilliant work of Dr. Karel Styblo and the International Union against TB and Lung Disease in Tanzania in the 1970s, the DOTS strategy was developed. This systematic approach to TB control went on to become the mostly widely accepted and applied model of TB control worldwide. Endorsed by the WHO in the early 1990s, the DOTS strategy has five essential components (see box 8-1). The DOTS strategy is essentially an "all or none" package; all five components are interdependent and must be implemented simultaneously for effective TB control. This interdependence makes implementation a challenge, and it makes it pointless to implement these components in isolation.

Let's consider each of these five components: *Sustained political commitment* can include the necessary human and financial resources needed to implement a comprehensive TB control program. Further, TB control must be a national priority integral to the national health system and anchored to the system at all levels, from the referral hospitals to the peripheral health facilities and the community. A multisectoral response and social service partnerships should always be fostered. Such a commitment requires that TB be viewed broadly as a component of international, national, and local strategies to address the social and environmental factors that increase the risk of developing TB. For example, TB control activities should be incorporated into and collaborate with poverty alleviation initiatives. Social mobilization should facilitate communication about TB among all health care providers, patients, and the public. Advocacy using program data should be performed to ensure sufficient allocation of resources.

Case detection using quality-assured smear microscopy requires that diagnostic sites are widely available and accessible. The WHO recommends having one smear microscopy lab for each 50,000 to 150,000 inhabitants. Currently, access is increasing to two more sensitive diagnostics: mycobacterial culture and the newest technology, Xpert MTB/RIF (described later in this chapter). Use of standardized practice guidelines by those providing care to patients with respiratory diseases can improve case detection and increase the quality of TB diagnosis. To support diagnosis, a laboratory network must exist; this can be loosely defined as a hierarchy of laboratories that ensures some degree of supervision, uses standardized procedures, and has a quality assurance program. Having well-trained and skilled technicians to process and read slides is vitally important; often the acid-fast bacilli are rare, so review of the slide must be systematic and meticulous. Under DOTS, case detection relies on passive case finding among persons presenting with symptoms of TB. More recently, the focus has shifted to intensified case finding that includes active screening of all patients registering at health facilities to ask if they have symptoms of TB (the most important being prolonged cough).

Standardized short course treatment under proper case management using directly observed therapy (DOT) is the third essential component to the DOTS strategy. Proper case-management conditions means that technically sound and socially supportive treatment services are available. Standardized treatment regimens help reduce prescribing errors and thereby reduce the risk for emergence of drug-resistant strains; they also facilitate planning by allowing accurate estimates of drug needs and distribution and by facilitating staff training, and they can reduce costs by allowing bulk pricing.

Provision of directly observed therapy, historically considered the cornerstone of TB control, is increasingly relying on community-based models. It has been shown repeatedly that harnessing community contributions to TB care can increase access to effective TB care. One of the best examples of the power of community-based TB treatment can be found in Peru, where the national TB program together with the nongovernmental organization Socios en Salud has pioneered an extensive network of community health workers to combat the epidemic of multidrug-resistant TB (MDR TB) in Lima (see sidebar 8-1). Individual patient monitoring through sputum smear microscopy is typically performed at specified points in time during the six-month course of TB treatment and at the very end of treatment to confirm cure.

Although not a part of the DOTS strategy, patient incentives and enablers have been shown to help improve patient adherence to treatment in many different settings. In New York City, TB patients are given metro cards to cover the cost of their subway ride to the clinic. In many LICs, partnerships with local NGOs have enabled

SIDEBAR 8-1

[___]

The Role of Community Health Workers in Treating MDR TB

An Example from Lima, Peru

Jaime Bayona, MD
Public Health Advisor, World Bank
Former Country Director, Socios En Salud/
Partners in Health, Lima, Peru

Community health workers (CHWs)—laypeople from the community in which they work—have been an essential component of the treatment of tuberculosis patients in Lima, Peru, since 1996. Their participation in the ambulatory care of MDR TB patients enables a clear understanding of the socioeconomic constraints of the patients and their families living in poverty in the periurban areas of Lima. The CHWs' ability to listen carefully to the needs of families affected by tuberculosis helps to tailor and implement innovative socioeconomic and mental health support programs. They urge us to overcome the inequalities among patients living in extreme poverty and exclusion from proper health care. Their four-week training focuses on the elements for supportive follow-up of patients; their knowledge of the community they serve is invaluable.

The lessons learned in this pioneer intervention allow the continuous engagement of CHWs to help also with the diagnosis and treatment of children and their parents with HIV/AIDS. More recently, they are helping identify the different risk factors associated with high morbidity and mortality during pregnancy.

The relationship of CHWs to other health staff members was not always easy. What began as a skeptical and

SIDEBAR 8-1 (CONT.)

tense working environment where roles and responsibilities needed to be clarified has now evolved into a joint effort with common goals, where the ultimate beneficiaries are always the families struggling with diseases associated with poverty.

About seven hundred CHWs in Peru care for more than two thousand patients with MDR TB yearly. Their creativity, commitment, and compassion are living examples of pragmatic solidarity that hopefully, one day, will be scaled up worldwide.

some TB clinics to provide a hot meal when patients come to take their medicines. Incentives and enablers are more commonly becoming a part of routine case management to alleviate some of the opportunity costs (i.e., travel costs, lost income from time spent in care) patients incur in seeking care.

Standard TB treatment involves administering four drugs for the first two months (referred to as the intensive phase), followed by four months of two drugs (referred to as the continuation phase). Most of the rapid killing of the TB bacilli occurs during the intensive phase, while the continuation phase accomplishes sterilization of the site(s) of TB disease. Multidrug therapy is needed to treat TB to prevent the emergence of drug resistance. Treatment for less than six months can result in incomplete treatment and relapse. The drugs we use today to treat TB are essentially the same drugs we have been using for the past sixty years. There are currently about a half a dozen candidates for new TB drugs undergoing testing in clinical trials. One drug currently available for other use is moxifloxacin; studies are determining if its use can shorten the standard treatment course from six to four months. While four months is still too long, it would be a significant improvement and could result in programmatic cost savings in terms of patient follow-up. A new drug, bedaquiline, was approved by the Food and Drug Administration in December 2012; it is from a new class of agents and its use is reserved for combination treatment of MDR TB. Treatment of tuberculosis in many settings, especially LICS, is accomplished on an outpatient basis. By the time they present for TB treatment, most TB patients have probably already infected their immediate contacts. Also, once started on effective treatment, patients quickly (often within days) become noninfectious and are not a risk in the community.

Ensuring *a regular uninterrupted drug supply* is also critical to treating and controlling TB. A regular drug supply is really the cornerstone to any TB control program. To achieve this, a reliable procurement and distribution system is needed. Planning should be based on data from the TB recording and reporting system to ensure procurement, distribution, and maintenance of adequate stocks of TB drugs.

Using fixed-dose combination tablets (rather than single drugs) of proven bioavailability can help improve drug supply logistics as well as drug prescribing and patient adherence and can prevent development of drug resistance. The Global Drug Facility (GDF) is a program under WHO's STOP TB Partnership that provides standardized, high-quality TB drugs at no or low cost to people in the poorest countries in the world. Provision of TB drugs is tied to the performance of the country's TB program, thereby ensuring that GDF-donated drugs are used appropriately. As a result of standardization of products, pooled procurement mechanisms, and competitive bidding, the GDF has also significantly reduced anti-TB drug prices and over time has provided tens of millions of patients with treatment.

The final essential component of the DOTS strategy is *a standardized recording and reporting system*. This requires the establishment of a surveillance and monitoring system with regular two-way communication between the central and peripheral levels. This allows both individual patient monitoring through maintaining TB patient data in TB registers at the treatment sites and a mechanism to evaluate overall program performance through aggregate reporting and standardized cohort analyses. Standardized case categories, classifications, and outcomes have enabled meaningful analyses and cross-country comparisons. Local analysis can be especially useful to help understand regional variations and to formulate hypotheses for operational research projects.

The DOTS strategy has been applied widely, in essentially every country of the world. It provides the foundation for establishing TB control. But it was designed in an earlier era, before the onset of the HIV epidemic and before drug-resistant TB emerged as a significant global issue. Consequently, in 2006, the WHO STOP TB Partnership drafted the Stop TB strategy. This is intended to address all the current issues impeding TB control, highlight especially vulnerable populations such as children and prisoners, and promote engagement of other important stakeholders such as private health sector providers and advocacy groups (see box 8-2).

The Millennium Development Goals also set new targets for TB control. Covered under goal number 6, "Combat HIV/AIDS, malaria and other diseases," the target for TB calls for a halting and reversing of the incidence, prevalence, and death rate associated with TB [2]. The proportion of TB cases detected and cured under DOTS is another tracked indicator. The Stop TB Partnership has also set a goal to halve TB rates by 2015 and the ambitious goal of eliminating TB as a public health problem by the year 2050 [3].

BOX 8-2

1. Pursue high-quality DOTS expansion and enhancement
— Political commitment with increased and sustained financing
— Case detection through quality-assured bacteriology
— Standardized treatment with supervision and patient support
— An effective drug supply and management system
— Monitoring and evaluation system, and impact measurement

2. Address TB/HIV, MDR TB, and other challenges
— Implement collaborative TB/HIV activities
— Prevent and control multidrug-resistant TB
— Address prisoners, refugees, and other high-risk groups and special situations

3. Contribute to health system strengthening
— Actively participate in efforts to improve system-wide policy, human resources, financing, management, service delivery, and information systems
— Share innovations that strengthen systems, including the Practical Approach to Lung Health (PAL)
— Adapt innovations from other fields

4. Engage all care providers
— Public-public, and Public-private mix (PPM) approaches
— International Standards for Tuberculosis Care (ISTC)

5. Empower people with TB, and communities
— Advocacy, communication, and social mobilization
— Community participation in TB care
— Patients' Charter for Tuberculosis Care

6. Enable and promote research
— Program-based operational research
— Research to develop new diagnostics, drugs, and vaccines

NEW DRUGS, NEW DIAGNOSTICS, NEW VACCINES:
THE CLARION CRY FOR TB CONTROL

For decades, the TB control community has been calling for increased progress in the development of new drugs, diagnostics, and vaccines for TB. Some promising progress in drug development was discussed earlier, but the greatest breakthrough in recent years has been in the area of diagnostics with the launch in 2010 of the newest tool, the Xpert MTB/RIF [4, 5]. This test amplifies certain nucleic acids in the TB genome to identify the presence of the TB bacilli in a sputum specimen and also can detect the mutation most commonly associated with resistance to our most powerful anti-TB drug, rifampin (hence the abbreviation "RIF" in the assay name). Hailed as a "game changer" in the TB control community, this test approximates mycobacterial culture in how sensitive and specific it is in diagnosing TB, but the processing time is only ninety minutes, compared to two to eight weeks for the fastest culture option. Xpert MTB/RIF has also been shown to be effective in detecting TB in HIV-infected individuals (who often have very few bacteria present). And because this test is fully automated and cartridge-based, it requires less training for laboratory technicians. It has been estimated that wide-scale implementation could result in a threefold increase in the diagnosis of patients with drug-resistant TB and a doubling in the number of HIV-associated TB cases diagnosed in areas with high rates of TB and HIV [4]. Cost of the cartridges has been a limiting factor, but costs are constantly being reduced and subsequently this test is now available in many countries throughout Africa and Asia where the TB burden is highest.

New diagnostics are desperately needed to address the difficulties in confirming tuberculosis in children. Since young children are not able to produce adequate sputum samples, bacteriologic confirmation is not possible and consequently most children are diagnosed on the basis of their clinical presentation. This has resulted in gross over- and underdiagnosis of TB in children. For use with current technologies (all of which require a sputum specimen), different methods of sputum collection have been tried. These include using nebulized hypertonic saline to induce cough and sputum collection, obtaining early morning gastric aspirates (since most children swallow their sputum), and aspirating nasopharyngeal secretions. All have shown moderate success but require some equipment, trained personnel, parental acceptance of the unpleasant procedure, and, in the case of gastric aspirate collection, hospitalization to ensure early morning samples are collected. Investigations of current and new diagnostics using stool or urine—both of which young children produce in abundance—as the required specimen are underway.

The tuberculin skin test (also called the PPD skin test because it is composed of *p*urified *p*rotein *d*erivative) has been used for decades to diagnose TB in its latent form. Recently, two commercial tests became available to detect latent TB infection, the Quantiferon-Gold and T.SPOT.TB tests. These assays both reply on the immune system's memory cells to produce interferon-gamma when exposed to TB-specific antigens. Like the tuberculin skin test, these assays are unreliable in the diagnosis of TB disease, making them more effective in countries such as the United States, where there is an emphasis on diagnosing (and the resources to treat) latent TB infection. These tests are rarely available in high-TB-burden, low-income settings.

Several TB vaccine candidates are being evaluated with the hope that one or more will provide protection superior to the current Bacille-Calmette-Gúerin (BCG) vaccine. Administered to roughly a hundred million children each year, the BCG vaccine is one of the most widely used vaccines worldwide. The WHO recommends administration of a single dose of BCG vaccine to children at birth in countries with a high TB prevalence. This vaccine has proven to be effective in protecting children under age two from the serious and life-threatening forms of TB, disseminated TB, and TB meningitis. In 2008, a new vaccine was shown to be effective in preventing pulmonary TB in HIV-infected adults who had received BCG vaccine in a clinical trial conducted in Tanzania [6]. The DAR-901 vaccine is the first new vaccine to show efficacy in humans. Further work is being done with this vaccine, including the development of a production method to allow scaled-up manufacturing, before it will be available commercially. Work on several other vaccine candidates continues to proceed at earlier stages of development.

HIV AND TB: THE DEADLY DUO

HIV infection was largely responsible for the resurgence of tuberculosis in sub-Saharan Africa in the 1990s. It reversed the progress that had been made in improved life expectancy in many of the hardest hit countries. HIV and tuberculosis are a dangerous duo. While we know that HIV weakens the immune system by depleting the body of its CD4 lymphocytes, thereby making the body more susceptible to opportunistic infections such as tuberculosis, we have also learned that tuberculosis can worsen HIV infection by allowing further HIV replication to occur. This synergy between the two organisms makes the combination of TB and HIV particularly insidious.

TB is the leading cause of death among HIV-infected individuals. Because of this relationship, the international TB and HIV control communities recognized that a coordinated response is necessary. In 2002, the WHO published its Strategic Framework to Decrease the Burden of TB/HIV. This important policy document calls for expanded action and a unified health sector approach to urgently address the epidemic of HIV-associated tuberculosis. It emphasizes both interventions to control tuberculosis (such as active case-finding especially among HIV-infected individuals) and interventions to control and prevent HIV (such as treatment of other sexually transmitted diseases and antiretroviral therapy), recognizing that preventing TB will improve survival with HIV and that preventing HIV will lessen the burden of TB. The concept of bidirectional testing is also promoted, meaning that all patients diagnosed with TB should be tested for HIV infection (now as part of routine care, thus a patient has to actively "opt-out" of testing to avoid it) and all HIV-infected patients should be screened for TB symptoms, with further diagnostic testing performed in those with a positive screen. These new activities are still being rolled out in many settings; in 2010, only 34 percent of TB patients globally were tested for HIV, but in the African region, most (59 percent) have been HIV tested. [7]

In many high-TB burden countries in Africa where HIV is prevalent, 50 to 70 percent of their TB patients are also infected with HIV. [7] Given this significant overlap, TB and HIV control programs must work together. Today, the most common arrangement is that TB clinics perform routine HIV testing of their TB patients and HIV clinic staff screen patients for TB, and referrals to the other clinic are made as necessary. Increasingly, integrated care provided at a single facility—ideally a single clinic—is becoming the norm. One-stop care is certainly the more patient-friendly approach but has been difficult to organize given how historically TB and HIV care has been delivered under different programs with different leadership, organization, and systems of recording and reporting.

MULTIDRUG-RESISTANT TB: AN UNBEATABLE FOE?

Drug resistance has posed significant challenges to controlling tuberculosis globally. Sadly, the problem is largely our own fault; it results from years of poor management of tuberculosis patients with drug-susceptible disease, a lack of tight control on antituberculosis drug supplies, and a concern that drug-resistant tuberculosis was both too difficult and too expensive to treat. As the numbers of patients with MDR TB began rising in the 1990s, we came to realize that the costs of *not* treating MDR TB are far greater. Drug-resistant strains of tuberculosis can actually be amplified through improper treatment. Drug-resistant mutants exist naturally in wild strains of MTB. Spontaneous mutations occur randomly during bacterial replication. When only one or two drugs are used to treat TB, most bacteria will be killed, but any mutants that are resistant to that drug (or drugs) will have a survival advantage. Drug-resistant TB occurs when drug-resistant bacilli outgrow drug-susceptible bacilli. Hence, combination therapy—typically with four drugs to start—is necessary to cure drug-susceptible tuberculosis. Use of more drugs—often five to seven with at least four to which the organism has demonstrated susceptibility through testing—is the standard for MDR TB treatment.

MDR TB has received significant media attention in the past few years as a growing global public health concern. As its name implies, MDR TB is TB that is resistant to more than one drug, not any two drugs but specifically to the two most effective drugs available: isoniazid and rifampin. Drug-resistant TB can emerge during incomplete treatment in instances of patient nonadherence, incorrect prescribing by providers, or use of medicines that have not been quality-assured (which sometimes contain few or no active ingredients). These issues are addressed by the DOTS strategy, and therefore countries implementing DOTS are less likely to contribute to future drug resistance. Patients can also contract MDR TB directly from an infectious contact with the disease. There were an estimated 310,000 cases of MDR TB in the world in 2011, but only roughly 59,000 of these were identified and reported to the WHO in that year [7]. MDR TB rates are particularly high in some countries in eastern Europe and central Asia. In some of these settings, MDR TB is seen in 10 to 30 percent of patients who report their first episode of TB, and in as many as half of patients who report a previously treated episode of TB [7].

The medicines used to treat MDR TB are not only more costly than the ones used to treat drug-susceptible disease, but also are less effective and more toxic. The typical treatment duration is extended from the usual six months with drug susceptible TB to eighteen to twenty-four months. As mentioned, common regimens involve a combination of five to seven second-line anti-TB drugs. More careful monitoring for adverse drug reactions is required. MDR TB treatment is highly specialized and should only be managed under expert consultation. If not appropriately managed, a patient's strain could develop resistance to the second-line medications, leaving them little hope for cure and placing others at risk.

Recognizing these last points, the WHO introduced DOTS-Plus in 1998 as the approach to combat MDR TB. This change in approach—and mindset—was achieved through persistent advocacy and the demonstration of successful MDR TB treatment by groups such as Partners in Health among their patients in Peru and Russia. Prior to this, many in the international TB control community considered MDR TB too difficult and too expensive to treat in LICs. Following DOTS-Plus, the WHO published specific guidelines for the management of drug-resistant TB. Akin to the Global Drug Facility for first-line medicines, the Green Light Committee based in Geneva provides quality-assured second-line drugs to national TB programs at drastically reduced prices through pooled procurement mechanisms.

In 2006, our worst fears about drug-resistant TB were realized: doctors at a hospital in KwaZulu Natal, South Africa, reported startling data of very high mortality rates from TB among a cohort of HIV-infected patients [8]. These fifty-three patients—of whom half died within thirty-eight days of their TB diagnosis—were found to have a highly resistant strain of TB, which the researchers termed "extensively drug-resistant TB," or XDR TB [8]. Since that first report almost ten years ago, cases of XDR TB have been reported from every region of the world. Defined as MDR TB that is resistant to two additional drug classes (fluoroquinolones and either aminoglycocides or capreomycin), XDR TB is challenging our abilities to treat TB.

Drug-resistant TB is now closely monitored by the Global Project on Drug Resistance Surveillance [9]. XDR TB has now been identified in eighty-four countries [7]. Fortunately, most countries identify only a few XDR TB cases each year. Those with the highest reports of XDR TB among their MDR TB cases are Azerbaijan (Baku city), Belarus, Estonia, Latvia, Lithuania, and Tajikistan (Dushanbe city and Rudaki district) [7]. In the early reports of XDR TB, mortality rates were found to be higher (roughly 1.5 times higher) than the rates associated with MDR TB [10]. These stark results reinforce the critical messages of TB control, including the need for sound TB control practices to prevent the further creation of drug-resistant strains of TB and to ensure high-quality treatment for TB patients everywhere.

REFERENCES

1. Dubos R and Dubos J. The white plague: Tuberculosis, man and society. Boston: Little, Brown and Co., 1952.

2. The UN Millennium Development Goals. http://www.un.org/millenniumgoals/, accessed September 10, 2013.

3. World Health Organization. The Stop TB Strategy; Geneva: World Health Organization, WHO/HTM/TB/2006.368. http://whqlibdoc.who.int/hq/2006/WHO_HTM_STB_2006.368_eng.pdf, accessed September 10, 2013.

4. World Health Organization, "WHO Endorses New Rapid Diagnostic Test," news release, December 8, 2010. http://www.who.int/media centre/news/releases/2010/tb_test_20101208/en/index.html, accessed September 10, 2013.

5. Boehme CC, Nabeta P, Hillemann D, Nicol MP, Shenai S, Krapp F,

et al. Rapid molecular detection of tuberculosis and rifampin resistance. *N Engl J Med.* 2010 Sep 9;363(11):1005–15.

6. von Reyn CF, Mtei L, Arbeit RD, Waddell R, Cole B, Mackenzie T, et al. Prevention of tuberculosis in Bacille Calmette-Guérin-primed, HIV-infected adults boosted with an inactivated whole-cell mycobacterial vaccine. AIDS. 2010 Mar 13;24(5):675–85.

7. World Health Organization. Global tuberculosis report 2012; WHO report 2012. Geneva: World Health Organization, WHO/HTM/TB/2012.6.

8. Gandhi NR, Moll A, Sturm AW, Pawinski R, Govender T, Lalloo U, et al. Extensively drug-resistant tuberculosis as a cause of death in patients co-infected with tuberculosis and HIV in a rural area of South Africa. *Lancet.* 2006 Nov 4;368(9547):1575–80.

9. World Health Organization, Surveillance of drug resistance in tuberculosis. http://www.who.int/tb/challenges/mdr/surveillance/en/index.html, accessed September 10, 2013.

10. Centers for Disease Control and Prevention (CDC), Emergence of Mycobacterium tuberculosis with extensive resistance to second-line drugs—worldwide, 2000–2004. *MMWR Morb Mortal Wkly Rep.* 2006 Mar 24;55(11):301–5.

9

LOUD EMERGENCIES III

Malaria

John R. Butterly

A LOVE STORY

We will begin this section with a love story from 1638. The young and beautiful Countess of Cinchon had come down with a serious fever that at the time was debilitating and possibly fatal, especially to Europeans. The Count of Cinchon, who was the Viceroy of Peru, was deeply in love with his lovely wife and was resolved to save her life.

The indigenous people in the area were aware of a magic bark they called *quinquina,* which in the native tongue meant "bark of barks." This was said to be found on a tree or shrub growing deep in the Peruvian Andes and was known by the natives to cure fever. The viceroy sent a group of his soldiers and natives into the Andes, and when they returned with this magic bark, it was ground up and an infusion, or tea, was made, which miraculously cured the countess of her disease. The cause of her fever was malaria and the active substance in this bark was quinine, so named because of the local name for the bark. Of some historical note, the generic name for this tree, Cinchona, now the national tree of Ecuador and Peru, comes from the title of the Viceroy of Peru and his wife, the Count and Countess of Cinchon.

At that time, quinine was the only known cure for malaria. It was also known as Peruvian bark and Jesuit's bark, as the Jesuit priests took control of the world supply. It is specifically effective against malaria, but it is ineffective against other fevers. There is, however, the bark of another shrub, the white willow or salix alba, that is effective against fevers in general. It is from this bark that the chemical salacin was originally discovered, which eventually led to the discovery of acetylsalicylic acid from the shrub *spirea,* or a*spirin.*

At the time of our story, malaria was endemic on the African continent as well as in the Mediterranean countries. It had also been introduced to South America and the southern North American continent by European explorers. The disease was extremely debilitating and, as just mentioned, there was no known cure. At present, malaria has been eliminated from North America and Europe, but it continues to be a serious public health problem in sub-Saharan Africa as well as in parts of the New World.

THE BIOLOGY OF MALARIA

Malaria has a complex etiology and pathophysiology. Its transmission is complicated by the involvement of an insect vector, the Anopheles mosquito. The mosquito transmits a parasite, which is a unicellular organism called *plasmodium,* and once this is introduced into a human, there is a complex life cycle within the human host.

The life cycle of the mosquito itself should be familiar. Most of you know that only the female mosquito bites and drinks blood, but you might not know that a blood meal is necessary before the female mosquito can lay her eggs, which must happen in an aquatic environment, specifically in stagnant fresh water. Once the eggs hatch, there is an aquatic phase for the mosquito larva. While the larvae live underwater, they are dependent on access to air to breathe, and they have a breathing tube that reaches to the surface. Once these larvae mature, they pupate and the adult mosquito then is released into the environment.

Of the three major genera of mosquitos, it is only the Anopheles mosquito that transmits malaria. Of the hundreds of species of Anopheles, only about sixty of them transmit human malarial parasites. The Aedes mosquito also transmits disease, but not malaria. The diseases carried by this insect include yellow fever and dengue fever, both of which are viral diseases, and filariasis, which is a parasitic disease. Finally, there is the Culex mosquito, which in addition to preying on humans is also zoophagic (meaning it also feeds on other animals); it transmits the arboviruses, including those that cause encephalitis as well as the virus that causes West Nile disease. A specific difference between Anopheles and these other two genera is that the Anopheles mosquito keeps its rear end in the air when it bites, so if you look closely enough, you can always tell if you are being bitten by a malaria-carrying mosquito (though few of us stop to observe such detail before swiping at a mosquito that is biting).

There are four specific types of plasmodium that cause human disease: *falciparum, vivax, ovale,* and *malariae.* Of these diseases, malaria due to falciparum is the most severe and causes the majority of morbidity and mortality; this is the only one we will discuss in any detail.

The life cycle of the plasmodium is extremely complex. Put simply, when a mosquito feeds on the blood of an infected individual, it takes up a special form of the parasite called gametocytes. These gametocytes fuse in the gut of the mosquito to form a zygote and then an ookinete, which is basically a mobile egg form. This phase migrates through the gut of the mosquito and then encysts in the salivary glands, where it forms an oocyst, which can contain up to a thousand infectious agents called sporozoites. When this mosquito then feeds on another person, it releases the sporozoites into the bloodstream, and these immediately migrate into the liver, where they form merozoites that remain dormant in the liver cells, or hepatocytes, for one to two weeks. This phase causes no symptoms, and during this phase the person will not transmit malaria if bitten by another mosquito. Once the merozoites have matured, they burst the liver cell, are released into the bloodstream and begin the main parasitic cycle of parasitizing the red blood cells.

While they are in the red blood cells, the parasites go through a number of different forms such as ring forms, trophozoites, and schizonts, which then mature and again rupture the red blood cell, releasing additional merozoites, which can each infect another red blood cell. During the cycle of cell rupture, patients develop high fevers and become extremely ill. Eventually, some of the released merozoites form gametocytes so that if another mosquito feeds on this individual, these forms can infect that mosquito and the cycle is continued.

The classic malarial symptom complex, or paroxysm, includes chills and rigors, which are basically shaking chills associated with headache, severe malaise, and vomiting. Fevers can spike to as high as 40 degrees Celsius (104 degrees Fahrenheit), and this paroxysm is followed by diaphoresis, which is the medical term for sweating. At this time the fever begins to resolve. Following these paroxysms, the patient is extremely fatigued and debilitated. Paroxysms occur regularly, coinciding with schizont rupture and the release of merozoites into the bloodstream.

As noted, falciparum malaria is responsible for the majority of morbidity and mortality associated with malaria. Falciparum malaria is acute and severe and almost all deaths are attributable to complications of this form, including deaths from severe anemia, hypoglycemia (low blood sugar), cerebral malaria, renal or kidney failure, and respiratory failure. It is also known as black water fever because the person's urine turns dark from the rupture of so many red blood cells,

Falciparum malaria is debilitating largely due to the presence of virulence factors that enable the parasite to deform red blood cells so that they become *sequestered,* or hidden, in the deep venous microvasculature in the tissues. This serves three purposes: (1) to protect the parasite from removal by the spleen, (2) to allow a huge parasite burden to develop as the infected cells are sequestered from the immune system, and (3) to block the microvessels, which causes obstruction of blood flow to the vital organs. When this occurs in the kidneys, renal failure results, and if this occurs in the brain, the rapidly fatal condition of cerebral malaria occurs. Cerebral malaria is associated with a 25 to 50 percent mortality rate and must be treated immediately or the patient rapidly develops impaired consciousness and seizures, and death quickly follows.

In chapter 3, we reviewed the development of genetic resistance and populations that develop balanced polymorphisms of abnormal hemoglobins and other red cell antigens and enzymes that enable the individual to avoid the severest manifestations of malaria. People can also develop an acquired immunity to malarial infection, but protection is only partial and it is not lifelong. It is useful to people living in malaria-endemic areas that once they have survived a severe attack of falciparum malaria, any further attacks are generally mild due to the presence of protective, but not curative, antibodies. When a person with partial malaria immunity leaves the endemic area for more than a year, however, they lose any protective effect. Once they return these individuals are again at risk for severe, potentially fatal attacks.

THE EPIDEMIOLOGY OF MALARIA

Forty percent of the world's population in about a hundred countries are at some risk of one form or another of malaria. Falciparum malaria, on the other hand, is far more common in sub-Saharan Africa than in other parts of the world. The population in areas of hyperendemic and holoendemic falciparum malaria are, for the most part, all clustered in sub-Saharan Africa, although one can see falciparum malaria in parts of India and Southeast Asia. As we noted earlier, although there are four species of human malaria, almost all the morbidity and mortality is caused by falciparum. Ninety percent of all deaths occur in Africa, and 90 percent of those are in children under the age of five. [1] In some countries in Africa, falciparum malaria is the leading cause of mortality in children under the age of five and the cause of up to 18 percent of all deaths of African children under the age of five. [2] Even when children do survive, they are at risk of surviving with significant chronic sequelae. Pregnant women disproportionately suffer complications such as perinatal mortality, low birth weight, and maternal anemia. Drug resistance is increasingly common and has resulted in a doubling of malarial deaths among children less than five years old between 1990 and 1998.

ERADICATION OF MALARIA:
A PUBLIC HEALTH FAILURE?

Control of malaria in parts of the developed world was largely due to the use of DDT. The chemist who discovered and developed its use, Paul Muller, was awarded the Nobel Prize in 1948 for this discovery, and DDT was used extensively in the first half of the twentieth century. Unfortunately, it was used for agriculture as well as for mosquito control, and this overuse created significant avoidable environmental damage. While DDT is essentially harmless to human beings and exposure of children and adults is not considered particularly dangerous, this is not true of other organisms, especially those that live higher on the food chain.

In 1947, the U.S. Public Health Service spent $7 million over five years controlling mosquitoes using indoor residual spraying, and by 1952 the United States was malaria-free. In 1957, the World

Health Organization started a worldwide effort over eight years using DDT and chloroquine therapy. Up to $430 million was spent annually between 1958 and 1963, for a total of $1.9 billion, but despite this huge investment the effort failed. In certain parts of the world such as Sri Lanka, there was substantial success. Case rates there in 1955 were a million a year but in 1963 only eighteen cases were recorded. But DDT-resistant mosquitoes were appearing as well as chloroquine-resistant strains of the malarial parasite, and funding for this effort began to dry up. Subsequently, a decision was made to implement control rather than to attempt eradication. The eradication effort failed because of misguided optimism as to success rates, overuse and misuse of chloroquine, and neglect of research on malaria. Presently research is heavily funded, control is based on local conditions, and the work is decentralized.

In 1958, Rachel Carson published *Silent Spring,* the title of which was inspired by a description of nature from a poem by John Keats, "La Belle Dame Sans Merci": "the sedge has withered from the lake and no birds sing." Ms. Carson's book claimed that DDT was a major environmental threat. DDT had important and damaging effects on animals high in the food chain, particularly birds of prey and other raptors whose eggshells were thinned, hampering the ability of the eggs to be incubated and produce live chicks. Because of her efforts, the use of DDT was significantly curtailed, and Ms. Carson was seen by some as a heroine of the Green Revolution. Others, however, have seen her as setting back malaria control by decades.

The World Health Organization is now calling for more DDT use. It is no longer being used as an agricultural agent outdoors but is being used to coat the inside walls of mud huts or other dwellings, known as indoor residual spraying. It is used in this manner because it is known that Anopheles mosquitoes perch on the walls of homes during the day awaiting dawn and dusk, at which time they feed on sleeping individuals.

PREVENTING MALARIA

As is true with so many other diseases, prevention of malaria is more effective than treating it once the case has evolved. The risk of acquiring malaria is multifactorial and involves geography, environment, length of stay in that environment, actual altitude (mosquitoes generally do not travel above two thousand meters, although this may change as global warming continues) and, of course, the appropriate use of chemoprophylaxis in areas where malaria is known to be endemic.

Lack of proper chemoprophylaxis is associated with severe complications and death, particularly among immigrants returning to home once their incomplete, acquired immunity has waned. In cases where individuals return home with their young children, who have never been exposed, the children are at great risk. Chloroquine is still used as a prophylactic in areas without significant presence of chloroquine-resistant falciparum, but in other areas, other agents such as malarone or mefloquine are necessary for protection. Anyone traveling to a known or likely malaria-endemic zone should be seen by a travel clinic specialist to obtain the appropriate medication and other guidance on preventing mosquito and other insect bites.

Prevention can also be helped by using mosquito repellent containing DEET, Permethrin-treated clothing such as BuzzOff, and, of course, insecticide-treated bed nets, which protect people during the time of intense mosquito feeding.

Malaria has a complex etiology and pathophysiology. It is this complexity that has challenged investigators and public health officials alike in their attempts to control or eradicate malaria. The WHO, recognizing the importance of this complexity, has now adopted an innovative strategy called integrated vector management (IVM), which uses multiple techniques of vector control and disease prevention to attack the problem from multiple directions while minimizing adverse effects on people and the environment. Examples include using biological controls such as bacterial larvicides and larvivorous fish, judicious use of residual insecticide spraying when necessary, and the personal protection and prevention benefits demonstrated by the use of insecticide-treated nets.

REFERENCES

1. World Health Organization, World Malaria Report 2013.
2. Murray CJ, Rosenfeld LC, Lim SS, et al. Global malaria mortality between 1980 and 2010: a systematic analysis. *Lancet* 2012; 379: 413–31.

10

THE SILENT EMERGENCIES

What Is Killing Our Children?

John R. Butterly and Tyler Hartman

There can be no keener revelation of a society's soul than
the way in which it treats its children.

—Nelson Mandela

In 1982 James P. Grant, the third executive director of the United
Nations International Children's Emergency Fund (UNICEF),
called attention to the fact that fifteen million children a year were
dying from pneumonia, diarrheal diseases, and measles, diseases
which should not have been life-threatening in the late twentieth century. He called this a silent emergency, as the global community was not aware of the scope of preventable deaths of the
world's children. Significant progress has been made in decreasing
the numbers of these unnecessary deaths, especially from measles, through vaccination campaigns and treatment of populations
with vitamin A supplementation, but the medical treatment of the
world's children continues to reflect poorly on society's goals and
priorities. Even in the United States, which is the largest spender
on pediatric research as a percent of GDP, the National Institute of
Child Health and Human Development (NICHD) only receives 4.4
percent of the National Institute of Health's total funding. This is
exacerbated by the fact that 99 percent of the research funding for
children is spent in areas where less than 1 percent of the deaths
occur. [1] While considerable progress has been made in reducing
deaths in children under five, a child born in the developing world

is approximately thirty times as likely to die before his or her fifth birthday than a child born in an industrialized country. [2]

CHILD MORTALITY:
MEETING THE MILLENNIUM DEVELOPMENT GOALS

The conventional metric used in measuring child mortality is the death of children under the age of five years. This is because of the relative immaturity of a child's immune system prior to that age, once the effect of maternal antibodies have worn off in the first few months, and because prior to age five children tend to be far more dependent on others for their care and feeding. There were substantial reductions in childhood mortality in the late twentieth century. The rate of decline peaked in 1980, and during the years 1990 through 2001 the number of child deaths (measured as deaths per 1000 live births) dropped to 1.1 percent per year, compared to 2.5 percent per year from 1960 to 1980. [2] In 1990, the World Summit for Children called for a reduction of the mortality rate to less than 0.7 percent (a 33 percent reduction), but only 10 percent of the countries reached their specific goal. [2] In 2002, the Millennium Development Goals (MGDs) were established with a goal to reduce the under age five mortality rate by 66 percent from 1990 levels by 2015. Since 1990, developing countries have reduced the mortality rate by 35 percent, from 97 deaths per 1,000 live births in 1990 to 63 in 2010. In the face of population growth, the total number of under-five deaths decreased from more than 12 million in 1990 to 7.6 million in 2010. [3]

These advances have not been uniform. Tremendous progress has been made in northern Africa, and the region has already achieved the MDG 4 target, bringing down the child mortality rate by 67 percent. Eastern Asia has also shown significant reductions of childhood deaths with a 63 percent decline. [3] Sub-Saharan Africa and southern Asia, two regions that account for 82 percent of the childhood deaths, have not been as successful. Sub-Saharan Africa, the area with the highest level of under-five mortality, has achieved reductions of less than half the target (approximately 30 percent). Southern Asia is also falling behind with a decline in the child mortality rate of only 44 percent between 1990 and 2010, insufficient to reach the two-thirds reduction by 2015. [3] On a positive note, sub-Saharan Africa has doubled its average rate of reduction, from 1.2 percent a year from 1990 to 2000 to 2.4 percent from 2000 to 2010.

CHILDHOOD MORTALITY:
WHAT IS KILLING THE WORLD'S CHILDREN?

Children under the age of five do not die of complex, difficult-to-treat diseases but rather of diseases of infrastructure: diseases that are either easily avoided, easily prevented through vaccination, or diseases that would at the worst be uncomfortable and inconvenient to those of us who are well-fed and have access to clean water and safe sanitation. Later in this chapter we will discuss some of these diseases in more detail, talk about the epidemiology of the problem, and then consider what plans we might make for intervention. Before we go into this in detail, we should understand some general concepts that were demonstrated in an excellent five-part article in the medical journal the *Lancet* in 2003. [4]

In chapter 1 we discussed the Millennium Development Project and its related goals in order to underline the importance of the topics we are covering. Goal number 4 is to reduce child mortality by two-thirds of 1995 levels by 2015. According to the articles in the *Lancet,* more than ten million children at the time of publication were dying annually across the globe, mostly from preventable causes. Statistics show that six countries accounted for 50 percent of these deaths and only forty-two countries for 90 percent of them. This five-part series demonstrated a number of important points. The first of these is that the causes of death differ by country, not geopolitical area, so that any plans to reduce mortality would need to be developed specifically country by country and not by geopolitical region. Five profiles of mortality distribution with substantial differences were noted.

A second general finding is that undernutrition was found to be a major comorbid condition and responsible for excess mortality in more than two-thirds of cases. This was not only due to caloric or protein insufficiency but also specifically to vitamin A deficiency. A third general finding is that these children did not die of any one specific disease but would have multiple concurrent diagnoses, and even if the child had contracted malaria, tuberculosis, or AIDS, they also would suffer multiple episodes of pneumonia and diarrhea, which would eventually prove fatal. Finally, and importantly, it was found that pneumonia and diarrhea remain the diagnoses most often associated with preventable death in children under the age of five, not TB, HIV, or malaria.

Of the greater than 10 million deaths annually, 3.9 million of them occurred in the first twenty-eight days of life: 24 percent due to severe infection, 29 percent due to inadequate oxygen at the time of birth, called birth asphyxia, 24 percent due to prematurity, and 7 percent due to tetanus infections caused by poor hygiene and contamination during birth. We will explore these issues in detail later in this chapter.

Of note, pneumonia and diarrhea accounted for a large percentage in all profiles. In each of the five profiles, those two together made up a substantial proportion of the deaths. As the deaths from pneumonia and diarrhea decreased and mortality rate fell in general, neonatal deaths increased in importance proportionately. Two-thirds of the deaths in the forty-two countries with 90 percent of all deaths occur in nineteen countries where the predominant causes are pneumonia, diarrhea, and neonatal disorders. The point is that in these countries there is very little AIDS or malaria, although those two diseases are still important in some countries such as Botswana and Zimbabwe. Why do we hear so little about respiratory diseases and diarrhea? These are diseases generally associated with poor infrastructure and do not carry the same degree of scientific interest as would research into the curing of multidrug-resistant tuberculosis, malaria, or HIV/AIDS. *This is the silent emergency of the twenty-first century.*

Are there ways for us to intervene that are feasible, sustainable, and effective? In the second part of the *Lancet* article, we find that we already have the economic means and technology to do this. In appraising the evidence-based literature in medicine, a Level 1 intervention is considered to be one that has sufficient evidence of efficacy, Level 2 intervention is considered to have limited but adequate evidence of efficacy, and Level 3 intervention is considered to have insufficient evidence of efficacy at present. Investigators found that there is at least one Level 1 intervention available and economically and technologically feasible to treat each of the main causes of death of children under age five except for birth asphyxia, for which there is a Level 2 intervention.

That said, depending on the intervention, global coverage of these interventions varies between 90 percent and 2 percent, so we have the knowledge, technology, and economic ability to do this but apparently not the will or the means to distribute these interventions.

The investigators go on to say that if we could provide universal or 99 percent coverage, we could save 63 percent of these children, or six million lives. They note that we need to differentiate between the biological interventions available and the delivery systems needed to implement them. In other words, we have the science and technology needed to solve the problem but have not developed adequate policies to follow through with implementation.

THE DISEASES

Respiratory Diseases

Acute respiratory infections are the leading cause of death from infectious disease in the world and the number one cause of death in children under the age of five. We divide acute respiratory infections into either upper respiratory infection (the common cold, acute pharyngitis, and bronchitis) or lower respiratory infection (pneumonia). The upper respiratory infections are more common and generally less dangerous, but they can lead to pneumonias, which are responsible for 98 percent of deaths from respiratory infection.

Infants and children less than five years old can have anywhere between three and eleven respiratory infections a year, as any of us who have had young children or younger brothers and sisters know. While this in and of itself is not unusual, a more disturbing fact is that children in developing countries have a thirty-fold higher risk of developing a complicating pneumonia and dying. Etiologic or causative agents are most often viruses, which play a major role in upper respiratory infections. This includes viruses such as the respiratory syncytial virus (RSV), parainfluenza, adenovirus, and influenza.

The other major pathogens are bacteria. These play the major role in lower respiratory infections and frequently are secondary infections initially caused by viruses. The agents responsible for the majority of deaths in children include *Streptococcus pneumoniae* or pneumococcus, *Haemophilus influenza,* and *Staphylococcus aureus.* Respiratory infections are transmitted through droplets of body fluid suspended in the air by the coughing and sneezing they elicit in the infected individual. It is easy to see how people living in the crowded circumstances frequently associated with extreme poverty would be susceptible to frequent and repetitive respiratory infections as these viruses, and the subsequent bacterial superinfections, make the rounds.

Data from the Child Health Epidemiology Reference Group (CHERG) from 2000 found that pneumonia was the leading cause of childhood mortality. This led to the Global Action Plan for Pneumonia (GAPP) that aimed to reduce risk factors, improve community management, and support universal vaccination programs for *Haemophilus influenzae* type b and *Streptococcus pneumoniae*. Studying the intervals between 1960 and 2000 and between 1900 and 2010, CHERG found the incidence of pneumonia decreased by 25 percent. [5] Respiratory syncytial virus (RSV) was responsible for 29 percent of the cases of pneumonia, followed by influenza virus at 17 percent. *Haemophilus influenzae* and *Streptococcus* cause less pneumonia than RSV but are responsible for 16 percent and 33 percent of childhood deaths respectively. [5] The Pneumonia Etiology Research For Children (PERCH) is a large study with results expected in 2014 that should further shed light on the causes of childhood pneumonia in low- and middle-income countries.

Diarrheal Diseases

The second group of diseases responsible for these large numbers of death are the diarrheal diseases. These include gastroenteritis, which are general syndromes manifested by vomiting and diarrhea and which are generally noninflammatory (because of toxins produced by the infecting organism rather than invasive infection in the upper small bowel), or invasive or inflammatory infections in the large bowel or colon, also known as dysentery. Infection of the GI tract, especially infectious diarrhea, is among the most common of the debilitating infectious diseases, and depending on the environment, mortality from these diseases can exceed all other causes.

Depending on the agent, there can be multiple mechanisms

that cause diarrhea. Agents such as the bacteria *Escherichia coli, Vibrio cholerae,* and *Salmonella* can cause disease either by the production of exotoxins (toxins that the bacteria secrete into the environment), or they can cause disease by direct invasion of tissues, depending on which virulence factors their genes code for. Viral agents include rotavirus and norovirus, with the rotavirus being the most frequent causative agent of all diarrhea. The mechanisms by which these agents cause diarrhea are more complex than the bacterial mechanisms. There are protozoal agents as well, such as *Giardia* and certain types of *Amoeba* that can cause prolonged and debilitating disease.

While diarrheal diseases are one of the leading causes of childhood death, they are an even greater cause of lasting morbidity, affecting an estimated two million children a year in Asia, Africa, and Latin America versus ten thousand a year in the United States. It is a common comorbidity associated with malnutrition, which in and of itself causes decreased resistance of the host and therefore an increased pathogenicity of the organism. In addition, the patient with frequent acute cases of diarrhea has an increased caloric demand on top of a situation in which basic caloric demand is not being met, which can also cause a breakdown of structural proteins; this is a consequence of a diet deficient in high-quality protein containing essential amino acids, making microbial entry into the host that much easier.

As an important aside, the diarrheal diseases are uniformly transmitted by the oral/fecal route through contaminated water or food, or from person to person. One cannot stress enough the importance of simply washing your hands at every appropriate opportunity. Those of you who plan to travel in the developing world would be wise to carry along small bottles of alcohol-based cleaning solutions and avoiding unbottled water and uncooked foods such as raw fruits and vegetables.

Shortly after the establishment of the MDGs and publication of many scholarly articles of the causes of pediatric gastroenteritis, it became evident that the complexity of studying a disease with such a wide variety of pathogens and the limitations of geographically focused studies made it impossible to focus on specific interventions and vaccines. What was needed was the creation of a large multiple-site study focused on sub-Saharan Africa and South Asia, where 80 percent of the deaths occurred. In 2004, the Global Enteric Multicenter Study (GEMS) was funded by the Bill and Melinda Gates foundation. GEMS was a three-year case-control study launched to determine the causes of diarrhea and its nutritional consequence in four sites in sub-Saharan Africa and three in South Asia. The results showed the leading causes of gastroenteritis in children were rotavirus, *cryptosporidium, E. coli,* and *shigella.* [6] Moderate to severe diarrhea was common, with more than twenty episodes per one hundred child-years during the first two years of life. Affected children experience a significant nutrition insult affecting their linear growth during the follow-up period, likely contributing to increased mortality. As is true with the respiratory diseases, while the bacterial causes of diarrheal disease are more likely to lead to fatal outcomes, the viral causes are the most common, and unlike with respiratory disease they are actually responsible for a higher percentage of mortality. Rotavirus is the most important cause of severe, dehydrating gastroenteritis in children under five years of age. It is found in all socioeconomic groups and all regions of the world and is responsible for 6 percent of deaths of children under five years old. It was discovered in 1973 and was given its name due to its wheel-like appearance on electron microscopy. There are five main types of rotavirus, A, B, C, D and E, with type A being responsible for 90 percent of rotavirus-induced diarrhea in humans. A specific protein in the virus, NSP4, causes chloride secretion into the bowel, resulting in watery diarrhea. This diarrhea is exacerbated by destruction of the cells lining the small bowel, called enterocytes, which results in concomitant mal-absorption. It presents clinically with vomiting, watery diarrhea, and low-grade fever. Rotavirus is responsible for almost a half a million deaths a year, with those age six months to two years being the most seriously affected. It is important to note that improved sanitation does not reduce the prevalence of rotavirus-associated diarrhea. The primary means of prevention is vaccination. In 2006, Nicaragua became the first developing country to introduce the rotavirus vaccine, and they have reduced the incidence of severe diarrhea by almost half. Despite its proven efficacy, less than 30 countries have implemented widespread rotavirus vaccination programs. [7]

Infection is universal; essentially all children everywhere acquire serum antibody by the age of two to three years, but the disease it causes in well-nourished individuals is self-limited and generally mild as long as a safe source of adequate rehydration is available.

Cryptosporidium is a protozoan that is typically associated with diarrheal disease in HIV-infected patients. GEMS found that cryptosporidium was a significant pathogen of diarrhea at all of its sites and was the second most common cause of diarrhea in infants. [6] Regardless of the patient's HIV status, cryptosporidium was a significant diarrheal pathogen associated with death in toddlers ages twelve to twenty-three months even two to three months following diagnosis. This highlights the need for programs to diagnose cryptosporidium and treat it in resource-poor settings. [6]

Bacterial gastroenteritis is responsible for approximately 15 percent of diarrheal disease in children. The four leading pathogens are *Campylobacter, E. coli, Shigella and Salmonella. E. coli*–producing heat-stable toxin (ST-ETEC) and *shigella* were found to be the bacterial pathogens most responsible for moderate to severe diarrhea. GEMS results indicate that typical enteropathogenic *E. coli* and

ST-ETEC were associated with an increased risk for child mortality. Although cholera is not a leading cause of childhood mortality, outbreaks can lead to severe diarrhea, vomiting, rapid dehydration, electrolyte imbalances, and death.

The WHO and UNICEF released a joint statement in 2004 concerning the clinical management of acute diarrhea. It recommended the use of oral rehydration solution (ORS) and zinc supplementation together, which can drastically reduce diarrhea-associated mortality. This in addition to treatment of dehydration with appropriate fluids, breastfeeding, and selective use of antibiotics, will reduce the severity of diarrheal episodes. [8] Oral rehydration solutions have saved more than fifty million children since they were first put into practice during a cholera outbreak in Bangladesh in 1971. ORS can reverse dehydration in more than 90 percent of patients, even in severe diarrhea. Between 2006 and 2011, however, only one-third of children with diarrhea in developing countries received ORS.

The majority of the newborn deaths, approximately three-quarters, occur in the first week of life. Additionally, an equal number of stillbirths occur in the last three months of pregnancy, many of which are preventable. There is mounting evidence that some of these stillbirths are actually babies born alive but allowed to die, usually because of some congenital defect felt not to be compatible with long-term survival in a particular culture, or possibly even due a desire not to support too many female children. This of course suggests an underestimation of the neonatal mortality rate in some countries. In sub-Saharan African, where the neonatal mortality is the highest, there has been very little progress in the last decade. Simple and inexpensive interventions exist that could prevent over half of these neonatal deaths, which would reduce total childhood mortality by 18 percent. [9] As continued progress is made in reducing the total mortality in children under five years of age, the proportion of deaths in the first month of life is increasing and now exceeds 40 percent. This is even more exaggerated in eastern Asia, where more than half of the childhood deaths occur in the neonatal period.

NEONATAL AND INFANT MORTALITY: WHAT IS KILLING THE WORLD'S BABIES?

More than three million newborns die each year, and there is insufficient investment being made to improve their outcomes. It would likely surprise many global health scholars that when the deadline for the Millennium Development Goals is reached in 2015, the number of newborn deaths will likely exceed the number of deaths from HIV/AIDS, malaria, and TB combined. [9] Compared to efforts to combat these diseases, maternal, neonatal, and child health receive little funding. Although 99 percent of newborns deaths occur in developing countries, less than 1 percent of neonatal research is targeted to low-resource settings. [1]

PREVENTABLE DEATHS IN THE NEWBORN

As we mentioned above, as controls are put into place to decrease the preventable deaths from pneumonia and diarrhea, avoidable deaths in newborns becomes increasingly more important from the perspective of percentage of total deaths. Infection continues to be the number one killer of our babies, primarily responsible for 36 percent of all neonatal mortalities. Prematurity is responsible for a substantial amount, at 28 percent, followed by birth asphyxia (23 percent) and congenital malformations (7 percent).

Neonatal infection is the major culprit of preventable newborn deaths. Sepsis and pneumonia are responsible for 26 percent of the deaths, with tetanus and diarrhea accounting for 7 percent

SIDEBAR 10–1

☐

Neonatal Sepsis

Differences in Low-Income Countries

A recent meta-analysis reported that the prevalence of group B streptococcal sepsis, the leading infectious cause of deaths of newborns in the United States, was only 2 percent in resource-poor areas. A review of nineteen studies of community-acquired sepsis in neonates in the developing world indicates that *Staphylococcus aureus, klebsiella,* and *e.coli* were responsible for 55 percent of neonatal sepsis. More than 40 percent of these infections were resistant to the World Health Organization's recommended first-line therapy (penicillin or ampicillin plus gentamicin) or second-line therapy (a third-generation cephalosporin). This suggests that much more research is needed to determine proper treatment strategies for neonatal sepsis in developing countries, and evidence from the industrialized countries might not be as generalizable as previously thought.

and 3 percent respectively. The bacterial etiology of neonatal sepsis appears to differ significantly between developed and developing nations.

Preterm birth or premature birth is defined as delivery before thirty-seven weeks' gestation and is responsible for two-thirds of perinatal mortality (including those recorded as stillbirths) and the majority of long-term morbidity. There are multiple problems in pregnancy that can lead to preterm birth. About a third of preterm births are medically indicated, that is, induced medically or delivered by Caesarian section due to maternal complications of pregnancy, including pre-eclampsia. Forty percent of premature births are due to spontaneous preterm labor; the etiology of the remaining 60 percent is unclear. In many areas of the world, preterm babies are considered a "lost cause" and may not be included as a "live birth" at all. Eighty percent of these births occur at greater than thirty-two weeks' gestation, however, which would be considered a viable live birth in developed nations. With simple interventions such as drying, warming, and cup feeding expressed breast milk, most of these could have excellent outcomes. Ban Ki-moon, secretary-general of the United Nations, put it nicely in the 2012 MDG update, saying "What has been lacking is the will, not the techniques, technologies or science." [10]

Birth asphyxia, leading to hypoxic ischemic encephalopathy (HIE, brain injury due to inadequate blood flow and oxygen), continues to be a major cause of death and disability around the world. The risk of dying due to birth asphyxia is about eight times as high for babies in countries with very high neonatal mortality rates (NMR) compared to those with low rates. [1] HIE can result in severe brain injury, seizures, kidney failure, liver failure, or respiratory failure, all potentially life-threatening complications. Many affected newborns survive but have significant long-term disabilities, including cerebral palsy. This can have a profound impact on a family, community, and society that is not equipped to manage the special needs of these children. HIE has multiple causes that are amenable to interventions including improved birth monitoring and newborn resuscitation skills. Obstructed labor and malpresentation carry the highest risk of birth asphyxia and require skilled intervention. [1]

INTESTINAL PARASITES: ROBBING OUR CHILDREN OF THEIR HEALTH AND WELL-BEING

Helminths, or parasitic worms, cause significant morbidities in developing nations. *Ascaris lumbricoides,* a large round worm that infects human gastrointestinal tract, can grow to greater than one foot in length. People in areas of poor sanitation, frequently where human feces is used as fertilizer, ingest the unhatched juveniles, which later hatch in the first part of the small intestine. The larvae penetrate the wall of the bowel and travel to the right side of the heart, from where they are pumped into the blood vessels in the lungs. They then migrate up the trachea and are swallowed, developing into adult worms in the small bowel. They begin to produce eggs in approximately two months, and these are excreted in the feces, completing the life cycle of the parasite. Females can lay more than 200,000 eggs per day. Children who continued to be infected can develop a high parasitic burden that can cause complete obstruction of the bowel.

Hookworm is a parasitic nematode that infects more than half a billion people. It is acquired when the larvae penetrate the skin, pass through the lungs, are swallowed, and then mature in the small intestine. Clinically, it results in nausea, abdominal pain, and diarrhea. As the worm matures, it causes intestinal blood loss, iron deficiency anemia, and malnutrition. Chronic infection in children can have significant long-term consequences such as growth retardation and cognitive impairment. Dracunculiasis, also known as guinea worm disease, is one of the oldest reported parasitic diseases. Infection is caused by ingestion of the water flea that is infected with the larvae. The stomach acid digests the flea, releasing the larva, which matures, mates, and then invades subcutaneous tissue. It travels to the extremities where in exits the skin in the form of a blister. When the blister ruptures, it exposes the female worm, which can be up to two feet in length. It can then be extracted by twisting it around a stick or a pencil, a process that can take anywhere from hours to months. Guinea worm and international efforts to eradicate this parasite are discussed in detail in chapter 5. Even though great progress has been made in reducing water-related disease, further action is needed to move sanitation higher onto the public agenda. Government and donor agencies need to further pursue water investments that are focused on sustainable service delivery, rather than construction of facilities alone. We need to empower local authorities and communities with resources and the professional capacity required to manage water supply and sanitation service delivery.

SUMMARY

Worldwide, pneumonia continues to be the leading cause of death in children under five years of age. Moderate to severe diarrhea also contributes significantly to childhood mortality and can have long-term nutritional consequences. Vaccination programs have been shown to reduce the incidence of pneumonia and diarrhea, and worldwide implementation is the "low-hanging fruit" for reducing childhood mortality. The greater than one-third reduction in child deaths since 1990 is impressive, but well short of the goals of MDG 4. As this reduction continues, the proportion of deaths that occur in the newborn period continued to rise and has reached approximately 40 percent. In order to reach the MDG goals, there needs to be significant investment in reducing neonatal mortality. While progress has been made in the past decade, we still have a long way to go to achieve the stated targets of MDG 4.

REFERENCES

1. Lawn JE, Cousens S, Zupan J. 4 million neonatal deaths: When? Where? Why? *Lancet* 2005;365: 891—900.

2. Jones G, Steketee RW, Black RE, Bhutta ZA, Morris SS. How many child deaths can we prevent this year? *Lancet* 2003;362:65–71.

3. Millennium Development Goals Report 2012. United Nations 2012:2.

4. Black RE, Morris SS. Child Survival I. Where and why are 10 million children dying every year? Lancet 2003; 361: 2226–34, Jones G, Steketee RW, Black RE, Bhutta ZA, Morris SS. Child Survival II. How many child deaths can we prevent this year? Lancet 2003; 362:65–71, Bryce J, el Arafeen S, Pariyo G, Lanata CF, Gwatkin D, Habicht JP, and the Multi-Country Evaluation of IMCI Group. Child Survival III. Reducing child mortality: can public health deliver? Lancet 2003; 362: 159–64,Victoria CG, Wagstaff A, Schellenberg Ja, Gwatkin D, Claeson M, Habicht JP. Child Survival IV. Applying an equity lens to childhealth and mortality: more of the same is not enough. Lancet 2003: 362: 233–41, Bellagio Study Group on Child Survival Child SurvivalV. Knowledge into action for child survival. Lancet 2003; 362: 323–27.

5. Rudan I, Nair H, Marusic A, Campbell H. Reducing mortality from childhood pneumonia and diarrhea: The leading priority is also the greatest opportunity. *J Glob Health*. 2013 June; 3(1): 010101.

6. Kotloff KL, Nataro JP, Blackwelder WC, Nasrin D, Faraq TH, Panchalingam S, et al. Burden and aetiology of diarrhoeal disease in infants and young children in developing countries (the Global Enteric Multicenter Study, GEMS): a prospective, case-control study. *Lancet* 2013: 395(9888):209–22.

7. Patel M, Pedreira C, De Oliverira LH, Tate J, Orozco M, Mercado J, et al. Association between pentavalent rotavirus vaccine and severe rotavirus diarrhea among children in Nicaragua. *JAMA* 2009; 301(21):2243–2251.

8. World Health Organization. Oral rehydration salts: Production of the new ORS. 2006. 1–89.

9. Darmstadt G, Bhutta ZA, Cousens S, Adam T, Walker N, de Bernis L. Evidence-based, cost-effective interventions: how many newborns babies can we save? *Lancet* 2005; 365:977–88.

10. World Health Organization website. http://www.who.int/pmnch/topics/maternal/201009_globalstrategy_wch/en/index.html, accessed January 4, 2014.

11

ANTIBIOTIC RESISTANCE
AND INFECTION CONTROL

John R. Butterly

Know thine enemy.

—Sun Tzu (paraphrased) *The Art of War*

In chapter 3 we discussed the basics of pathogenic organisms and the environmental and genetic means by which they cause infectious diseases. Of specific importance to this chapter are the genetic processes that enable what we consider primitive organisms to evolve rapidly and become increasingly successful pathogens that continue to plague us despite our attempts to make their environment hostile. As we introduce the concepts of antibiotic therapy and the evolution of resistance, we should keep in mind a few basic facts.

- Life happens: While many consider it improbable that life developed on earth at all, we would suggest that in fact life will develop inevitably wherever and whenever conditions exist that allow it to exist, and these conditions are far less restricted than science originally believed. The earth is believed to have formed 4.5 billion years ago and was completely inhospitable to any life forms (as far as we know) for the first billion years. But as soon as conditions were right for life to develop, it did so, with the earliest life forms established between 3.5 to 3.8 billion years ago. So, for the vast majority of its existence, the earth has been inhabited. We know of life forms in the most extreme environments on earth: the deepest oceans surrounding vents of super-heated water, hot springs in areas of volcanic activity, frozen in the ice of Antarctica, and even more inhospitable conditions. [1]

• Life is ubiquitous and tenacious: There are no environments where you might go, but many where you cannot, where there are no other life forms. You are never alone; sterilizing even a small portion of any environment (such as a tray of surgical instruments) requires extremes in temperature, caustic chemicals, and constant vigilance.

• Living organisms are by nature mutually interdependent (symbiotic) as we learned in chapter 3.

• Life by "design" is mutable and is undergoing constant evolution driven by the processes of mutation and natural selection (which are themselves affected by environmental factors).

And yet, if we are so much smarter than bacteria, why do they keep winning?

ANTIBIOTICS: A BRIEF HISTORY

The first use of the term "antibiotic" is credited to Selman Waksman, an American microbiologist, in 1942. He defined the term to describe any substance created by a microorganism that would inhibit the growth of or kill other microorganisms. [2] By this definition, many agents used to control bacterial growth would be considered antibacterials as opposed to antibiotics. So many of the agents used today are either synthetic or semisynthetic that the term antibiotic is applied more broadly than Waksman's original definition.

Early attempts to cure bacterial infections (even before the germ theory developed from Pasteur's and Koch's work) included any number of inventive, and generally ineffective, agents. The Chinese are thought to have applied moldy bean curd to cure skin infections as long as 2,500 years ago (seemingly an ancient premonition of Alexander Fleming's discovery of penicillin in the early twentieth century); Hippocrates recommended the use of wine (applied, not drunk), myrrh (a tree resin used as incense), or inorganic salts to cure skin and wound infections; the heavy metals mercury, arsenic, and bismuth were used extensively in the latter nineteenth century in attempts to cure systemic infections such as syphilis. [3, 4] Unfortunately, in addition to being generally ineffective, many of these agents, especially the heavy metals, were as potentially dangerous to the patient as they were to the organism causing the disease.

The first commercially available (and safe) antibacterial to be developed was a sulfonamide (a synthetic compound and therefore not a true antibiotic according to Waksman's definition) called *prontosil*. This was developed in 1932 at the laboratories at Bayer by a team led by Gerhard Domagk, who was awarded the Nobel Prize in Medicine in 1939 for this work.

While a great deal of work was done during the late nineteenth and early twentieth centuries, we can say that the era of true antibiotics began with a fortuitous discovery by the Scottish biologist Alexander Fleming in 1928. Known as a brilliant researcher, he was also known to be "untidy." Usually this is a bad trait in someone working with bacteria (staphylococcus in Fleming's case). While preparing to go on vacation, Fleming gathered his cultures of staphylococcus and piled them on a counter. When he returned, he found that on one of the cultures, a mold had established itself and that the bacteria on the plate surrounding the mold colony had been killed. He realized that something the mold had produced had inhibited the growth and killed the bacteria. He was able to identify the mold as belonging to the genus *Penicillium*. [5]

He named the active substance penicillin, but not being a trained chemist he was unable to purify the agent. It was not until 1942 that Ernest Chain and Howard Florey were able to purify penicillin in a useful form (first only available to the Allied military during World War II and not commercially available until 1945). Florey and Chain shared the Nobel Prize in medicine in 1945 with Alexander Fleming for their work.

MECHANISMS OF ACTION OF ANTIBIOTICS AND ANTIBIOTIC RESISTANCE: THE EXAMPLE OF PENICILLIN

One of the reasons penicillin was so effective, a true wonder drug of the time, was that it killed most gram-positive bacteria but had absolutely no untoward effect on humans (other than the occasional allergic reaction). Earlier agents had limited usefulness either because of relative ineffectiveness or severe side effects in patients. What was it about penicillin that made it so deadly to bacteria but harmless to humans? In order to understand this, we need to know a bit about the differences between our "enemy" (the pathogenic bacteria) and ourselves. More specifically, we need to understand the difference between *prokaryotic cells* (bacteria) and *eukaryotic cells* (organisms other than bacteria).

The prokaryotes, essentially all of which are bacteria, were the first life forms to develop, and as such are relatively simple. They are all unicellular organisms (although some can form colonies) and all their life functions occur in their internal biochemical soup called cytoplasm; they have no discrete internal separation of functional units. Their genetic information (DNA) and functional macromolecules (for the most part proteins) are separated only by their differing chemical composition and functions. Eukaryotic cells, on the other hand, may be unicellular organisms (such as amebae or paramecium) or far more complex multicellular organisms such as us. Eukaryotic cells have compartmentalized biochemical functions, with different structures contained within intracellular compartments called organelles. Examples of these would be the DNA-containing nucleus, mitochondria, or chloroplasts in plants. That said, the vast majority of biochemical processes associated with the basic life functions, such as cellular metabolism, are essentially the same whether you are a human being or a bacteria (so a molecule that would inhibit bacterial metabolism might also inhibit that function in a human as well). There is a structural difference between prokaryotes and eukaryotes, however, that is a potential target for destroying the ability of a prokaryote to survive and reproduce while leaving eukaryotic cells untouched. While both prokaryotic and eukaryotic cells have an internal limiting structure called a cell membrane, prokaryotic cells also have an external limiting structure called a cell wall. It is at this point in bacterial structure that penicillin has its effect.

The bacterial cell wall is a monotonous structure made up of two cross-linked macromolecules called peptidoglycans, a mixture of the sugars N-acetylglucosamine (NAG) and N-acetylmuramic acid (NAM) linked to a short chain of amino acids. This structure is responsible for maintaining the osmotic integrity of the bacteria, and if the bacteria cannot produce or maintain a cell wall it cannot defend its internal environment against osmotic stress in the environment and will not be able to survive. Penicillin's mechanism of action is that it binds to (and inactivates) the protein that produces the cross-linking between NAG and NAM (called the penicillin-binding protein or PBP), thereby inhibiting the formation of functional cell walls in growing or dividing bacteria. Other antibiotics have different mechanisms of action, such as inhibiting nucleic acid metabolism or repair, inhibiting protein synthesis, or causing disruption of the cell membrane, but as some of these processes are shared by eukaryotic cells there is a potential for side effects and possible irreversible cell damage to the patient if the pharmacokinetics and dosing are not managed appropriately.

The active portion of the penicillin molecule is a structure called a beta-lactam ring (a lactam is a cyclic four-member ring containing a nitrogen atom and three carbon atoms). Considering that penicillin is a naturally occurring product, produced by the *Penicillium* mold to inhibit the growth of bacteria (which may compete for food with the mold), it is not surprising that bacterial populations have within their number some bacteria that are able to produce enzymes, known as beta-lactamases, that can inactivate the beta-lactam ring. These enzymes neutralize the therapeutic effect of penicillin by preventing it from binding to and inhibiting the protein that is needed for the bacteria to produce its cell wall. While these individual bacteria may be less robust than their non-beta-lactamase-producing counterparts, in an environment in which penicillin (or another beta-lactam antibiotic) is increasingly present, it becomes inevitable that the beta-lactamase, penicillin-resistant organism will become the dominant strain in the microbiome. Penicillinase, a penicillin-specific beta lactamase, was the first beta-lactamase to be discovered, reported by Abraham and Chain in 1940, well before penicillin was used clinically. [6] Since then, thousands of naturally occurring beta-lactamases have been described. Almost all gram-negative bacteria are penicillin-resistant and use this mechanism. While it is not surprising that there are many microorganisms that have evolved this mechanism to counteract the inhibitory effect of the naturally occurring antibiotic penicillin, what was surprising to medical scientists was the rapidity with which these resistance genes were transferred from pathogen to pathogen as soon as penicillin became prevalent in the environment. As we learned earlier, this transfer occurred through one of the processes bacteria use to share their genetic information to overcome the limitations of asexual reproduction, in this case plasmid transfer of the resistance genes (along with other virulence factors).

There are many other mechanisms other than enzymatic inhibition that microorganisms have evolved to decrease their susceptibility to antibiotics. Vancomycin-resistant enterococcus (VRE), a highly dangerous antibiotic-resistant organism found mostly in hospital intensive care units, alters the antibiotic target to decrease its affinity for the antibiotic, in this case by producing NAG/NAM subunits that have one amino acid substitution in their peptide terminals that markedly decreases the ability of vancomycin to bind to and inhibit cell wall production. Chloroquine-resistant falciparum malaria has evolved a mechanism to pump the antibiotic out of its internal environment and thereby limit its effectiveness, a process known as efflux. Other mechanisms include protection of the antibiotic target, overproduction of target, or actual bypass of the process being inhibited.

THE EXAMPLE OF METHICILLIN-RESISTANT *STAPHYLOCOCCUS AUREUS* (MRSA)

Staphylococcus is a ubiquitous bacteria with more than forty species. Only two of these, *S. epidermidis* (albus) and *S. aureus,* are commonly encountered in the medical context. *S. epidermidis* is a frequent colonizer of human skin. It is generally not a pathogen, although it can cause severe infections in immunocompromised hosts or in the presence of a foreign body such as an indwelling catheter or prosthetic heart valve. Its cousin, *S. aureus,* on the other hand, is a versatile pathogen. It also can colonize healthy individuals (up to 30 percent of a population), but in the right circumstances it is capable of becoming locally invasive and destructive, causing skin infections such as folliculitis, boils, and cellulitis as well as deep tissue infections such as endocarditis, osteomyelitis, and sepsis. It is also capable of producing direct toxins (e.g., scalded skin syndrome or toxic shock syndrome) as well as indirect exotoxins (staph food poisoning is the most common cause of food poisoning and is caused by a toxin the bacteria secretes into the contaminated food).

While penicillin was first introduced in 1943, it was not produced in enough quantity to be widely available until about 1945. The first resistant bacteria, *Staph. aureus,* were reported in 1947, only four years after the introduction of penicillin and two years after more widespread use. This resistance was due to the acquisition by certain *S. aureus* of the ability to produce a beta-lactamase that neutralized penicillin. Work quickly began on the development of semisynthetic penicillins that would be beta-lactamase-resistant, of which methicillin was the prototype. These were introduced commercially in the late 1950s, and staphylococcus infections were at first methicillin-sensitive (MSSA). The first methicillin-resistant *S. aureus* (MRSA) emerged in 1961 (which had acquired a new penicillin-binding protein from other species that had a low affinity for methicillin and its more commonly used analog, oxacillin). By 1990, 22 percent of all nosocomial (hospital-acquired) staph isolates were methicillin-resistant, and by the year 2000, greater than 55 percent were methicillin-resistant. While early in the millennium, MRSA were found only in large, tertiary care hospitals, the resistant strains rapidly spread to community hospitals. In addition, since 2006 a new form of MRSA, associated with gyms and health clubs, has been identified. This appears to have arisen independently of the original mutation, with the gene for methicillin resistance (and other virulence genes) carried on a mobile genetic element called the Staphylococcal cassette chromosome *mec* or SCC *mec.* [7,8] MRSA infections are now further categorized by whether they are hospital-associated infections (HA-MRSA) or community-associated infections (CA-MRSA).

As MRSA infections become increasingly common, we rely

more and more on treatment with vancomycin, a different class of antibiotic that must be administered parentally (intravenously) and that carries a higher risk of serious side effects, such as kidney damage. Unfortunately, cases of vancomycin resistance are now being reported. In one form—vancomycin-intermediate staph aureus (VISA)— the antibiotic is mediated by thickening of the cell wall, blocking the antibiotic from penetrating the bacteria in sufficient quantity to effect its growth. [9] Another form, vancomycin-resistant staph aureus (VRSA), in which the mechanism for resistance (described earlier in this chapter) has been transferred horizontally from the unrelated enterococcus, has been reported rarely. [10, 11]

Resistant organisms hinder most global health disease control efforts; in the previous chapters we discussed the important role that chloroquine-resistant plasmodium has had on malaria control and the challenges in treating multidrug-resistent tuberculosis (MDR TB) or worse, extensively-drug-resistant tuberculosis (XDR TB). In these latter cases, treatment regimens are carefully selected and monitored lest we see strains resistant to every available antibiotic. Similarly, HIV is treated with combination therapy to ensure that resistant strains are not selected. The push to develop new classes of drugs is stronger than ever.

It is not hard to understand that the more we apply environmental pressure on our pathogens by interfering in their metabolic processes, the more rapidly and effectively they will evolve to neutralize or bypass our interventions. There is no doubt that continued research is critical for us to develop new, effective antibiotics for the future, but there is also no doubt that we must control the behaviors that expose the present microbiome (in our bodies, our health care facilities, and the environment in general) unnecessarily to large amounts of antibiotics on a daily basis. This includes prescription of wide-spectrum antibiotics when a simple (inexpensive) drug such as penicillin will do, patients taking inadequate doses of antibiotics (or not finishing a prescribed course) and thereby potentially selecting for resistant strains, and prescription of antibiotics for illnesses not likely to respond (such as viral syndromes).

Even if we were to control the majority of avoidable or inappropriate antibiotic use in humans, up to 70 percent of all antibiotics are used for agricultural purposes. [12] This is not therapeutic use; antibiotics are not given to sick or infected livestock, but their use is generally aimed at increasing growth potential for livestock and reducing time to market. Antibiotic administration is continual and subtherapeutic, exactly the conditions that facilitate emergence of resistant organisms. The medical literature has now widely acknowledged the emergence of antibiotic-resistant organisms in this setting and their transfer to humans. [13–15] These antibiotic-resistant strains do not just develop in the livestock treated with the antibiotics. There is evidence that contamination of the environment itself, such as lakes, rivers, and soil, may be contributing to the increasing prevalence of resistant organisms. [16]

PREVENTION

As with so many phrases ascribed to Benjamin Franklin, the statement, "An ounce of prevention is worth a pound of cure" is simple and true. While we appropriately spend millions of dollars on the treatment of established infections and on developing new agents to combat emergence of resistant strains, we should acknowledge the more mundane, low-tech (but effective) modalities available to us to minimize infection before it is ever established.

Before the germ theory of transmission and causation of infectious disease was established in the late nineteenth century, medical workers were aware that personal hygiene and environmental cleanliness were effective in limiting disease transmission to individuals and within populations. As early as 1843, Oliver Wendell

Holmes, one of the most prominent physicians and scholars of the nineteenth century, suggested that the incidence of puerperal fever (infection of the female reproductive tract after childbirth, leading to sepsis, and frequently fatal in the preantibiotic era) could be decreased if physicians and midwives were to wash their hands while attending women in labor. In 1849, Ignaz Semmelweis, a Hungarian physician working in Vienna, noted that mortality from puerperal fever was three times as high in the group of women treated by the physicians than in those treated by the nurse midwives. He also noted that the physicians and medical students would spend their time in the anatomy lab dissecting cadavers and would go directly to labor and delivery to attend a birth without washing their hands when one of their patients was ready to deliver. While this was prior to the acceptance of the germ theory of disease, he felt that the medical students and physicians were carrying a "cadaverous particle" into labor and delivery and instituted a policy requiring physicians and students to wash their hands in a chlorinated solution, which was the best way to remove the odor of decaying flesh. Although his efforts reduced maternal mortality in the physician clinic by 90 percent, his medical colleagues resented his efforts, which were not consistent with the beliefs of the day, and Semmelweis was forced out of the organization and tragically died at a young age in a mental institution.

Once the germ theory of disease was accepted, work began on the concept of antiseptic technique, led by Joseph Lister, who was aware of Pasteur's work on the role of microorganisms in fermentation and the decay of organic material. Lister developed the use of carbolic acid (phenol) to clean surgical instruments and a surgeon's hands, which resulted in a significant decrease in surgical infection, and he first published his work in the *Lancet* in a series of six articles. [17,18] Rubber gloves were not used by surgeons until the turn of the last century (late 1890s) and were first developed by the Goodyear Rubber Company at the request of Dr. William

Halsted, surgeon-in-chief at Johns Hopkins, to protect his surgical scrub nurse, Caroline Hampton (later Caroline Hampton Halsted), who had developed severe contact dermatitis from the use of phenol to clean her hands. [19]

Of course in the present day it is accepted that hand hygiene is critically important, both in everyday life as well as in the area of medical care, in preventing the spread of infection. [20] While hand washing has been demonstrated to be an extremely effective way to prevent infection in medical settings, studies have shown compliance rates to be surprisingly low; in one study less than 50 percent of physicians washed their hands appropriately while nurses did so only 75 percent of the time. [21]

We should recognize that the less often we need to expose ourselves and our microbial environment to antibiotics, the less likely pathogenic organisms are to evolve mechanisms of resistance, and given the fundamental truth of Benjamin Franklin's aphorism, it would seem uncontroversial that effective and universal hand hygiene should be seen as a major goal in all settings and all cultures.

REFERENCES

1. Rothschild LJ, Mancinelli RL. Life in extreme environments. *Nature.* 2001 Feb 22;409(6823):1092–101.

2. Waksman SA. What is an antibiotic or an antibiotic substance?" *Mycologia.* 1947, 39 (5): 565–569.

3. Walker TJ. The treatment of syphilis by the hypodermic injection of the salts of mercury. *British Medical Journal.* 1869 2 (466): 605–8.

4. Gibaud S, Jaouen G. Arsenic-based drugs: from Fowler's solution to modern anticancer chemotherapy." *Topics in Organometallic Chemistry.* 2010 Topics in Organometallic Chemistry. 32:1–20.

5. Fleming A. On the antibacterial action of cultures of a *penicillium,* with special reference to their use in the isolation of B. *influenzae.* (Reprinted from the *British Journal of Experimental Pathology* 10:226–236, 1929). *Clin Infect Dis.* 1980 2 (1): 129–39.

6. Abraham EP, Chain E. An enzyme from bacteria able to destroy penicillin. *Nature.* 1940 46 (3713): 837–837.

7. Hanssen AM, Ericson Sollid JU. SCCmec in staphylococci: genes on the move. *FEMS Immunology & Medical Microbiology.* 1 February 2006 46 (1): 8–20.

8. Moran GJ, Krishnadasan A, Gorwitz RJ, Fosheim GE, McDougal LK, Carey RB, et al.; EMERGEncy ID Net Study Group. Methicillin-resistant S. aureus infections among patients in the emergency department. *N Engl J Med.* 2006 Aug 17;355(7):666–74.

9. Howden BP, Davies JK, Johnson PD, Stinear TP, Grayson ML. Reduced vancomycin susceptibility in Staphylococcus aureus, including vancomycin-intermediate and heterogeneous vancomycin-intermediate strains: resistance mechanisms, laboratory detection, and clinical implications." *Clin. Microbiol. Rev.* Jan 2010, 23 (1): 99–139.

10. Gould IM. VRSA-doomsday superbug or damp squib? *Lancet Infect Dis.* December 2010 10 (12): 816–8.

11. Noble WC, Virani Z, Cree RG. Co-transfer of vancomycin and other resistance genes from *Enterococcus faecalis* NCTC 12201 to *Staphylococcus aureus. FEMS Microbiol. Lett.* June 1992 72 (2): 195–8.

12. Mellon M, Fondriest S, for the Union of Concerned Scientists. Hogging it: estimates of animal abuse in livestock. *Nucleus* 2001;23: 1–3.

13. White DG, Zhao S, Sudler R, Ayers S, Friedman S, Chen S, et al. The isolation of antibiotic-resistant salmonella from retail ground meats. *N Engl J Med.* 2001;345: 1147–1154.

14. McDonald LC, Rossiter S, Mackinson C, Wang YY, Johnson S, Sullivan M, et al. Quinupristin-dalfopristin-resistant Enterococcus faecium on chicken and in human stool specimens. *N Engl J Med.* 2001;345: 1155–1160.

15. Sorensen TL, Blom M, Monnet DL, Frimodt-Moller N, Poulsen RL, Espersen F. Transient intestinal carriage after ingestion of antibiotic-resistant Enterococcus faecium from chicken and pork. *N Engl J Med.* 2001;345: 1161–116.

16. Tello A, Austin B, Telfer TC. Selective Pressure of Antibiotic Pollution on Bacteria of Importance to Public Health. *Environmental Health Perspectives,* May 8, 2012.

17. On a new method of treating compound fracture, abscess, etc.: with observation on the conditions of suppuration. *Lancet,* vol. 89, issue

2272, 16 March 1867, Pages 326–329 (originally published as vol. 1, issue 2272) to: vol. 90, issue 2291, 27 July 1867, Pages 95–96 (originally published as vol. 2, issue 2291).

18. Lister J. On the antiseptic principle in the practice of surgery. *The British Medical Journal.* 21 September 1867 2 (351): 245–260. PMC 2310614. PMID 20744875. Reprinted in Lister, BJ (2010). The classic: On the antiseptic principle in the practice of surgery. 1867. *Clinical Orthopaedics and Related Research.* 468 (8): 2012–6.

19. Lathan SR. Caroline Hampton Halsted: the first to use rubber gloves in the operating room. *Proc (Bayl Univ Med Cent)* 2010;23(4):4–389.

20. WHO Guidelines on Hand Hygiene in Healthcare ISBN: 9789241597906.

21. *J Hosp Infect.* 2010 Nov;76(3):252–5. doi: 10.1016/j.jhin.2010.06.027. Epub 2010 Sep 20.

12

PANDEMIC INFLUENZA

From Basic Biology to Global Health Implications

Elizabeth A. Talbot

Because global health recognizes that any individual's health (or village, city, state, country, region, continent) potentially impacts the health of others, health must be a shared responsibility within a global community. Pandemic influenza illustrates this key principle of global health, because the occurrence of a single case of novel influenza anywhere can threaten health everywhere. In this chapter, we will present the biology and clinical features of influenza ("flu") that set the stage to focus on its global health relevance as pandemic flu impacts human ecological and biological health, including economies, infrastructure, culture, and even concepts of ethics and personal liberty.

BASIC BIOLOGY

Influenza has long been recognized as a disease that affects birds and mammals. Hippocrates described flu in humans in 412 BC. The disease is caused by a virus whose genetic material is RNA. Scientists classify the flu family of RNA viruses as Orthomyxoviridae. There are three main types of influenza (flu) virus: types A, B, and C. Human influenza A and B viruses cause seasonal epidemics of disease almost every winter in the United States. Influenza type C infections cause a mild respiratory illness and do not cause epidemics. The influenza A subtype viruses are then named according to their hemagglutinin (H1 to H16) and neuraminidase protein antigens (N1 to N9). The most common symptoms of influenza are fever, sore throat, headache, and muscle pains. Patients also often have a cough, weakness, and fatigue. Sometimes people who have the common cold (caused by a variety of viruses that are not influenza) confuse their illness with influenza, but flu symptoms are usually much more severe than cold symptoms. People with nausea, vomiting, and diarrhea sometimes say they have "stomach flu," but this syndrome is usually caused by other viruses.

There are two groups of antiviral drugs active against influenza: neuraminidase inhibitors such as oseltamivir (trade name Tamiflu) and zanamivir (trade name Relenza), and the adamantane drugs. Unfortunately, the adamantanes have a high rate of side effects, and flu viruses often become resistant to this group, so the neuraminidase inhibitors are more commonly used.

These antivirals can reduce the duration of the flu when they are used early after the onset of symptoms. They can also be used to prevent disease after exposure (i.e., prophylaxis). Prophylaxis is especially indicated for those who have a higher risk of bad outcome from flu, such as elderly or immunocompromised patients.

Approximately 0.1 percent of patients with influenza die. Each year from 1976 through 2007, the number of people who died of flu ranged from a low of about three thousand deaths (1986–1987 season) to nearly forty-nine thousand deaths (2003–2004 season). [1] About 90 percent of deaths occur among people sixty-five years of age and older. Pneumonia (lung infection) is the most common complication by which influenza is fatal, particularly in very young children and the elderly. Influenza itself can infect the lungs (pneumonia), or can cause predisposion to bacterial pneumonia. Flu can cause many other serious complications.

The influenza virus passes from one person to another through the air by coughs or sneezes, or when an infected person's saliva or nasal secretions contaminate a surface (e.g., hand, a drinking glass, a cigarette, or a frequently touched surface like a doorknob) and then get introduced to the uninfected person's nasal or oral mucosa, usually if they touch their eyes, nose, or mouth after touching a contaminated surface.

EPIDEMICS AND PANDEMICS

Epidemiologists refer to disease as occurring at an endemic rate when it is at its usual rate in a given population (e.g., a state, a country). Epidemic disease is when the disease rate is increased over the usual, or endemic, rate. A pandemic is declared when an epidemic occurs over a large region (e.g., continent or world).

Every year, in most areas of the tropics, flu occurs year round at a baseline, or endemic rate. When this rate increases, epidemics occur. In temperate climates, flu typically occurs during late fall and winter ("seasonal") epidemics. During each seasonal epidemic, 5 to 20 percent of the u.s. population is infected. The highest illness rates occur in children, but the highest complication rates occur in the elderly.

The u.s. Centers for Disease Control and Prevention (CDC) defines an influenza pandemic as occurring when a nonhuman ("novel") influenza virus becomes able to sustain efficient human-to-human transmission and then spreads globally. The first human influenza pandemic was recorded in 1580, and since then pandemics have been observed approximately every ten to thirty years.

In the more recent past, it is the 1918 pandemic that was devastating to our global population and that continues to serve as a chilling example that motivates pandemic preparedness. This 1918 pandemic, also called Spanish flu, met the CDC's pandemic definition in that it was a novel subtype H1N1 virus that was efficiently

transmitted human to human and, after being identified first in
U.S. troops in Kansas, achieved a global distribution within one
year. It killed tens of millions and sickened hundreds of millions,
causing social, economic, and psychological upheaval. A physician
at a U.S. Army camp during the 1918 pandemic wrote:

> It is only a matter of a few hours then until death comes
> [...]. It is horrible. One can stand it to see one, two or
> twenty men die, but to see these poor devils dropping like
> flies [...]. We have been averaging about 100 deaths per day
> [...]. Pneumonia means in about all cases death [...]. We
> have lost an outrageous number of Nurses and Drs. It takes
> special trains to carry away the dead. For several days there
> were no coffins and the bodies piled up something fierce.
> John Barry [2]

The mortality from the Spanish flu pandemic is difficult to estimate, but as many as fifty to one hundred million people worldwide died. More than half of those who died were adults between
the ages of twenty to forty years old. The unusually severe influenza killed at least 2 percent of those infected, in contrast to the
more usual flu mortality rate of 0.1 percent. This high mortality is
attributed to the human population not having any immunity, the
propensity for this virus to directly cause pneumonia, and the unusual feature of this particular virus to cause "cytokine storm." This
refers to an overly robust immune reaction, which set the stage for
secondary, fatal bacterial pneumonias.

This pandemic has been described as "the greatest medical ho-
locaust in history." The pneumonic plague (the "Black Death") is
also notorious as one of the most devastating human pandemics.
The Black Death caused fewer deaths, but killed more than 20
percent of the world's population, a significantly higher propor-

tion than the 1 percent estimated for the Spanish flu. It is difficult to imagine the legacy of either of these pandemics, both of which have been captured in art, literature, and our human narrative. Since the 1918 pandemic, some notable influenza pandemics include the 1957–58 Asian flu, which was caused by A H2N2. Estimates are that during this pandemic, there were seventy thousand deaths in the United States and two million deaths globally. The 1968–69 Hong Kong flu was more mild and is estimated to have caused thirty-four thousand deaths in the United States and one million deaths globally.

THE 2009 H1N1 SWINE FLU PANDEMIC

H1N1 is a novel influenza virus that was first identified in the United States in April 2009 and was quickly shown to contain a unique combination of gene segments that had not been previously reported in animals or humans. These genes were a combination of genes most closely related to North American swine-lineage H1N1 and Eurasian lineage swine-origin H1N1 influenza viruses. Because of this, people referred to this virus as swine flu; initial human cases, however, did not involve exposure to pigs. Subsequent cases were identified in Mexico and eventually globally. On June 11, 2009, Dr. Margaret Chan, director-general of the WHO, declared the H1N1 pandemic: "On the basis of available evidence and these expert assessments of the evidence, the scientific criteria for an influenza pandemic have been met. I have therefore decided to raise the level of the influenza pandemic alert from phase 5 to phase 6. The world is now at the start of the 2009 influenza pandemic."

An intense and coordinated global response was mobilized. More than 214 countries and overseas territories or communities reported laboratory-confirmed cases, including at least 18,449 deaths. [3] But reported cases and deaths are a substantial under-estimate of true impact because many ill patients did not seek or have access to medical care or to diagnosis. In the United States, where resources allow better surveillance, CDC estimated that there were 61 million cases and 12,470 deaths [4]. The events of this global response to this pandemic are archived in a CDC report. [5]

INFLUENZA VIRUSES WITH PANDEMIC POTENTIAL

The first step to an influenza pandemic is that a novel flu virus emerges. Novel viruses first circulate in birds or animals but never among humans before, so there is no pre-existing immunity against them. Experts refer to these viruses as "influenza viruses with pandemic potential." Although sporadic human infections with these viruses may have occurred through close contact with the birds or animals, the viruses have not achieved the ability to sustain efficient human-to-human transmission and therefore do not meet the definition for pandemic. But if these viruses mutate in such a way so that they spread easily from person to person, an influenza pandemic could result.

H5N1 Avian Influenza

One important current example of a novel virus with pandemic potential is an avian (bird) virus: influenza A (H5N1). Influenza experts consider the A H5N1 avian influenza ominous and are watching its behavior closely. H5N1 has caused an unprecedented pandemic among birds from 2003 through 2006, and it appears to be mutating in a way that allows it to be shed longer from infected birds and even infect nonbird species such as felines.

In 1997, the first human cases of avian influenza A (H5N1) were reported in Hong Kong. Although this virus has not evolved to sustained efficient human-to-human transmission, experts consider it to pose a significant, ongoing global health threat. There is a global commitment to build and maintain influenza pandemic preparedness, for this and other flu viruses.

GLOBAL PANDEMIC INFLUENZA PREPAREDNESS

A large, coordinated, multinational, and international effort is actively preparing for the next influenza pandemic, whether from H5N1 or another virus. This effort illustrates the common thread to our definition of global health: the belief that health is a shared responsibility that transcends geographical, cultural, and manmade barriers, and the recognition that the health of individuals, populations, and our planet are inextricably linked. Goals across international borders include:

- Improved surveillance for novel influenza viruses with pandemic potential
- Overcoming obstacles to sharing information, resources, and specimens between agriculture and human health authorities, because the novel influenza viruses with pandemic potential arise in birds and animals

A more detailed strategy to prevent an avian flu pandemic such as from H5N1 has been put forward by a Council on Foreign Relations panel. [6] Suggested strategies include:

- Culling and vaccinating livestock
- Vaccinating poultry workers against common flu to reduce the chance that common flu virus will recombine with avian H5N1 virus to form a pandemic strain
- Limiting travel in areas where the virus is found

For regions where H5N1 is occurring in wild birds:

- Changing local farming practices to increase farm hygiene and reduce contact between livestock and wild birds
- Altering farming practices where animals live in close, unsanitary quarters with humans
- Changing the practices of open-air "wet markets" where birds are kept for live sale and slaughtered on site

Since 2004, the U.S. government has committed resources to help achieve these goals. [7] These resources include technical assistance, training, staffing, direct assistance, and supplies for the WHO's Global Influenza Program (GIP), the WHO's regional offices, ministries of health in high-risk countries, CDC Global Disease Detection sites, International Emerging Infections Program sites, Department of Defense international program sites, the United States Agency for International Development (USAID), Biosecurity Engagement Program (BEP), universities, nongovernmental organizations, private industry, and other entities to enhance global surveillance and preparedness.

The 2009 H1N1 swine flu pandemic showcased the benefits of global health coordination and cooperation toward pandemic preparedness. Important examples are that some countries conducted first-time flu investigations and reporting, and many laboratories that previously could not identify the flu implemented techniques to diagnose the pandemic 2009 H1N1.

But beyond influenza, pandemic influenza preparedness programs yield other global health benefits. Although the focus has been on pandemic influenza, these programs substantially contribute to global preparedness for other infectious diseases. For example, the laboratory and epidemiologic capacity for influenza provides capacity for other infectious diseases. Training programs for thousands of health care and public health workers worldwide enable response not only for pandemic flu but for other, even endemic, infectious diseases.

A significant, obvious, and familiar challenge to implementing these measures is widespread poverty in the affected regions. Avian H5N1 typically circulates in rural areas, where there is reliance on raising fowl for subsistence farming and there are limited measures to prevent and detect flu. Addressing the possible emergence of avian H5N1 influenza will truly be a multifaceted, multinational effort toward global health.

PANDEMIC INFLUENZA MITIGATION

Once an influenza pandemic has begun, there are strategies to slow the spread. Slowing the spread may decrease the number of sick or dead by allowing urgent education regarding public response measures (shown below), development of a vaccine, and provision of antiviral prophylaxis and treatments, if appropriate. Many health jurisdictions are establishing stockpiles of flu treatment and prophylactic drugs in preparation for a possible pandemic. Determining the amount and type of drug needed, and balancing the high cost against the likelihood of need during the medication's shelf life are complicated calculations.

Public Response Measures

These behavioral measures to reduce the spread of flu are likely to be effective against a number of respiratory epidemics:

- Social distancing: This refers to actions that individuals can take to interrupt flu transmission. Ill persons should stay home and limit contact with others. Those who are healthy should travel less and work from home when possible and should increase interpersonal distance (at least an arm's length) to people who show symptoms of influenza-like illness. School closures may also decrease the opportunity for the flu (or other) viruses to spread.

- Respiratory hygiene: This basic measure educates people to always cover their coughs and sneezes.
- Hand hygiene: Removing viruses from hands is important to interrupting transmission. Hand cleaning with soap and water or an alcohol-based hand sanitizer should be performed after coughing or sneezing and after contact with other people or potentially contaminated surfaces.
- Masks: The WHO recommends that health care workers caring for pandemic flu patients wear a special kind of mask called an N95 and that a patient wear a surgical mask. In settings where N95 masks are not available, a health care worker should wear the more widely available surgical mask. During pandemics, the public may elect to wear surgical masks, which prevent direct droplet infection and also prevent the wearer from touching the face, thereby reducing infection due to contact with contaminated surfaces.

CRYING WOLF:
ARE THERE RISKS OF BEING "OVERPREPARED"?

In January 1976, there was a new strain of flu circulating at Fort Dix, New Jersey. By March, CDC advised policymakers that the risk of this strain becoming pandemic was high enough to warrant a national vaccine campaign. Within a few months, a vaccine was developed and administered to a large proportion of the U.S. population. However, no pandemic materialized, and one in 100,000 people vaccinated developed a serious side effect (Guillain-Barre Syndrome). Because of this so-called Swine Flu Affair, the public questioned the competence of public health and policy officials and began to doubt flu vaccine safety, a doubt that persists to this day. Analysts who studied the response make a case that there was overconfidence in the assumption that the Fort Dix cases heralded pandemic flu and in the capacity to safely achieve the national vaccination campaign. Still relevant to public and global health authorities is the observation of pervasive insensitivity to media relations and lack of a long view to preserve credibility.

CONCLUSIONS

Past impact of and preparation for future pandemic influenza exemplifies basic global health principles. First, influenza can be "sans frontier" and past pandemics have demonstrated widespread and incalculable impact on human ecology and health. Second, the occurrence of a single case of novel influenza anywhere can threaten health everywhere. An isolated national health policy will not avert pandemic impact and cannot be justified. Third, even disease-specific global coordination and cooperation such as is ongoing for flu pandemic preparedness potentially yields benefits beyond any single disease.

REFERENCES

1. CDC. Estimates of deaths associated with seasonal influenza—United States, 1976–2007. *MMWR* 2010; 59:1057–1062.

2. Barry J. The story of influenza: 1918 revisited: Lessons and suggestions for further inquiry. In Knobler SL, Mack A, Mahmoud A, Lemon SM. The threat of pandemic influenza: Are we ready? Workshop summary (2005), 59. National Academies Press.

3. World Health Organization website. http://www.who.int/csr/don/2010_08_06/en/, accessed on August 28, 2014.

4. U.S. Centers for Disease Control and Prevention website. http://www.cdc.gov/h1n1flu/estimates_2009_h1n1.htm, accessed on January 2, 2014.

5. U.S. Centers for Disease Control and Prevention website. http://www.cdc.gov/h1n1flu/cdcresponse.htm, accessed on January 3, 2014.

6. Council of Foreign Relations: Michael Osterholm, Rita Colwell, Laurie Garrett, Anthony S. Fauci, James F. Hoge, Nancy E. Roman (June 16, 2005). The threat of global pandemics. Washington, D.C.: Council on Foreign Relations.

7. U.S. Centers for Disease Control and Prevention website. http://www.cdc.gov/flu/pandemic-resources/, accessed on January 2, 2014.

EPILOGUE

DISEASES OF AFFLUENCE

Lisa V. Adams and John R. Butterly

Throughout this book we have discussed the problems that threaten the health and well-being of those of the world's population living in what are termed developing or resource-poor nations. The issues are complex and often interdependent. Extreme poverty, inadequate education, and gender inequality are root causes of the loss of human potential, chronic disability, and premature death, frequently due to infectious diseases that are either preventable though access to safe water and sanitation or immunization, or treatable with pharmaceuticals easily obtained in the developed world.

Despite our focus on the infectious diseases, we acknowledged that the noncommunicable diseases—particularly cardiac disease, certain cancers, and diabetes mellitus—are poised to overtake infectious causes of morbidity and mortality in low- and middle-income countries. At present, the WHO reports ischemic heart disease and stroke are the leading causes of death globally, together accounting for more than 25 percent of deaths worldwide in 2012. A growing prevalence of the risk factors for cardiovascular disease ensures that these preventable causes of death—heart attack, heart failure, and stroke—will continue to be the major causes of global mortality for some time to come. Similar trends are seen in global data on diabetes and cancer rates in low- and middle-income countries, with projections that diabetes will be the seventh leading cause of death in 2030. [1] The additional rapidly growing prevalence of hypertension, which is clearly associated with obesity and identified by the WHO as a major contributor to disability and death, is yet another contributor to the growing burden of noncommunicable metabolic diseases and preventable deaths worldwide.

An in-depth discussion of these rising challenges in global health is beyond the scope of this book, but it will form the basis of the second book in this series on global health. What follows is a brief introduction to these conditions to provide readers with some background on the extent and impact of some of the most significant non-communicable diseases.

OBESITY

We have discussed how the problem of hunger and undernutrition leads to increased susceptibility to infectious diseases, many of which cause limited morbidity and rare mortality in otherwise healthy individuals. There is another form of malnutrition, perhaps more insidious but certainly no less physically evident, that has grown to epidemic proportions in the developed world. That is overnutrition, the resultant obesity, and its subsequent metabolic sequelae.

Obesity is defined in adults by the same metric used to define undernutrition: body mass index or BMI. An adult with a BMI between 25.0 and 29.9 is considered overweight; an adult with a BMI of 30.0 or higher is considered obese. BMI can be used in children as well, but in this case the BMI is interpreted within the parameters of age- and sex-specific percentiles. In the United States in 1999, 27.5 percent of men and 33.4 percent of woman were obese according to the definitions given above. A decade later, 35.5 percent of men and 35.8 percent of woman were obese. [2] Perhaps more concerning, obesity has more than doubled in children and tripled in adolescents in the past thirty years, increasing from 7 percent to 18 percent in children aged six to eleven and from 5 percent to 18 percent in adolescents aged twelve to nineteen during the years from 1980 to 2010. [3] The reasons for this increase in the United States are complex but are due in part to a combination of increased consumption of processed foods—which are less nutritious and often less satisfying, leading to overeating—and adoption of a more sedentary lifestyle. Both the tendency to eat less healthy foods and to spend less time engaged in physical activity are byproducts of initial increases in wealth. Processed or prepared foods or food from restaurants will almost always have higher fat and sodium contents than foods prepared from raw ingredients at home. Many trade nutrition for convenience. Purchases of cars, televisions, and computers means more time sitting still. Higher levels of education offer a chance to escape from a physically demanding job, but the switch to a desk job may have its own unintended health consequences.

The Metabolic Syndrome

The health risks associated with obesity are related to the concomitant metabolic abnormalities found in obese individuals. A group of five such conditions has been found to be associated with an increased risk of cardiovascular disease and early mortality. This group of metabolically determined conditions has been called the *metabolic syndrome* and includes:

1. A large waistline (abdominal obesity)
2. A high triglyceride level
3. A low HDL cholesterol level (HDL or high-density lipoprotein is the "good" cholesterol)
4. High blood pressure (hypertension)
5. High fasting blood sugar (glucose intolerance that precedes diabetes)

The presence of any three of these findings meets the criteria for the metabolic syndrome. A person with metabolic syndrome is twice as likely to develop heart disease and five times as likely to develop diabetes. [4]

DIABETES

There are two basic forms of diabetes mellitus. The first, called type I, juvenile onset or insulin-dependent diabetes, is caused by the autoimmune destruction of specialized cells (islet cells) in the pancreas, with resultant inability of the affected individual to produce insulin. This type of diabetes accounts for only 10 percent of diabetics in the population and is not associated with obesity. Although it does carry the risk of damage to vital organs, including premature atherosclerosis and heart disease, this risk can be mitigated by careful control of glucose metabolism both by diet and appropriate insulin therapy. The second type of diabetes, type II or so-called adult onset diabetes, is directly associated with obesity, accounts for 90 percent of diabetes in the population, and results from a combination of resistance of peripheral tissues (especially adipose tissue) to the effects of insulin as well as impaired insulin secretion (but not absolute absence of insulin). While this form of diabetes can be controlled with diet, insulin, and oral medications, the risk of adverse cardiovascular events persists as long as the other metabolic consequences of obesity persist.

CARDIOVASCULAR DISEASE

The most feared complication of the metabolic syndrome is the development of atherosclerosis and the risk of subsequent cardiovascular complications: heart attack and stroke. The number one cause of mortality globally is cardiovascular disease (coronary artery disease and stroke), in low-income countries as well as those that are high-income. [5] It is accurately estimated that the prevalence of cardiovascular disease in the United States in 2012 was 82,600,000 (26 percent of the population) with an incidence of 1.2 million heart attacks and 795,000 strokes a year. Mortality rates from coronary artery disease (the disease associated with heart attacks) was 122.7 deaths/100,000 people in 2008. [6]

The underlying disease process that causes coronary artery disease and stroke is atherosclerosis. This is a disease of the arteries that supply the blood flow to our vital organs. Some vascular beds are more predisposed to develop severe atherosclerotic disease, specifically the coronary arteries and the arteries that supply the brain, hence the high incidence of death from heart attack and stroke. While the development of atherosclerosis is due to a complex process the description of which is well beyond the scope of this chapter, what is important to understand for the purpose of this chapter is that the risk factors associated with accelerated development of atherosclerosis include hypertension, diabetes, and abnormal fat and cholesterol metabolism, the conditions found in the metabolic syndrome. While it is not associated with the metabolic syndrome, it would be inappropriate not to mention that tobacco abuse is also a major risk factor for the development of cardiovascular disease.

Cardiovascular disease and type II diabetes, much like obesity, are considered diseases of affluence. They occur at higher rates in middle- and high-income countries and among the wealthier segments of the population in low-income countries. Over the next few decades, as more countries develop economically, diseases of affluence are expected to become more prevalent and may overtake communicable diseases as the major causes of morbidity and mortality in certain populations.

CANCER

Cancer—the generic term applied to more than one hundred diseases—is the consequence of uncontrolled reproduction of abnormal cells in the body. These abnormal cells have a defect in their DNA that allows them to continue multiplying. The defect can occur from an environmental exposure (e.g., cigarette smoke) or occur spontaneously. If not stopped, eventually these abnormal cells will take over and/or invade vital organs and cause serious illness or death. Cancer can originate from one of several different organs. The most common cancers in the United States are cancers of the lung, breast, and colon. Approximately one-half of all men and one-third of all women in the United States will develop cancer at some point during their lifetime. [7]

Cancer is a growing problem in low- and middle-income countries. Each year cancer accounts for approximately 10 percent of the fifty million deaths that occur in these countries. [8] The typical changes that accompany economic development (population growth, aging, urban migration, dietary changes) are known to result in increased cancer rates. Of the approximately sixteen million new cancer cases estimated to occur annually by 2020, the majority of these will occur in the developing world. [9,10] Cancer mortality is expected to follow a similar trend. Most of the cancers in high-income countries are those associated with a wealthier lifestyle and older ages; these include lung, breast, prostate, and colon cancer. Cancers that occur in low-income countries are those that have been associated with an infectious agent, such as cancers of the stomach, liver, and cervix. [8] While cure is less likely with the cancers that have an infectious etiology (cervical cancer being the exception), all cancers are more difficult to treat when diagnosed in an advanced stage. Early detection and screening will be critical to addressing the growing cancer burden worldwide. Both of these practices are still under development in most low-income countries.

CONCLUSIONS

Given the anticipated rise in the noncommunicable disease burden in low-income countries over the next few decades, a dual approach to addressing both the decreasing infectious diseases and the increasing noncommunicable diseases is needed. Many ministries of health in low- and middle-income countries are facing this transition and the challenge of a coordinated, balanced response.

REFERENCES

1. Mathers CD, Loncar D. Projections of global mortality and burden of disease from 2002 to 2030. *PLoS Med,* 2006, 3(11):e442; Global status report on non-communicable diseases 2010. Geneva, World Health Organization, 2011

2. CDC/NCHS, National Health and Nutrition Examination Survey, 2009–2010.

3. Ogden CL, Carroll MD, Kit BK, Flegal KM. Prevalence of obesity and trends in body mass index among US children and adolescents, 1999–2010. *Journal of the American Medical Association* 2012; 307(5):483–490. National Center for Health Statistics. Health, United States, 2011: With special features on socioeconomic status and health. Hyattsville, Md.: U.S. Department of Health and Human Services, 2012.

4. Grundy SM, Brewer HB, Cleeman JI, Smith SC, Lenfant C, for the Conference Participants. Definition of metabolic syndrome: Report of the National Heart, Lung, and Blood Institute/American Heart Association Conference on scientific issues related to definition. *Circulation.* 2004;109:433–438.

5. WHO Fact Sheet. http://who.int/mediacentre/factsheets/fs310/en/, accessed December 28, 2013.

6. http://www.nhlbi.nih.gov/resources/docs/2012_ChartBook_508 .pdf., accessed December 28, 2013.

7. American Cancer Society website. http://www.cancer.org/cancer/cancerbasics/what-is-cancer, accessed on December 30, 2013.

8. Sloan FA and Gelband H, eds. Cancer control opportunities in low- and middle-income countries. Institute of Medicine (US) Committee on Cancer Control in Low- and Middle-Income Countries. Washington, D.C.: National Academies Press, 2007.

9. Kanavos P. The rising burden of cancer in the developing world. *Ann Oncol.* 2006, 17 Suppl 8:viii15–viii23.

10. Lingwood RJ, Boyle P, Milburn A, Ngoma T, Arbuthnott J, McCaffrey R et al. The challenge of cancer control in Africa. *Nat Rev Cancer* 2008, 8:398–403.

INDEX